BYE BYE NORMAL
HELLO EXCEPTIONAL

BYE BYE NORMAL HELLO EXCEPTIONAL

Living a Life of Less Stress and More Energy!

SHAWNA CALE

Dedication

Mom

Thank you for always being there for me. You have always loved me, encouraged me, and supported me in what I have chosen to do. I love you!

Kevin

Thank you for loving me and our children unconditionally on this rollercoaster ride of life. I am the luckiest woman to love a man like you!

Ryan

The moment I saw you and became a mom, I felt a connection I had never felt before. I am so proud of the man you have become. I love you!

Emily

I always dreamed of having a beautiful little girl just like you. You are one of the kindest and loving women I know. I love you!

Bryce

You make me smile every day and have brought our family so much joy. Thank you for being such a sweet and loving son. I love you!

My Many Friends

Thank you for walking this life with me and being there when I needed a friend. Your love and support helped me grow and become the woman I am today. I appreciate and love every one of you. I am here for you.

Sunshyne

God knew I needed someone in my life that's strengths were my weaknesses. He knew I needed someone to keep me accountable to myself and to my dreams. He knew I needed someone to bring a smile to my face when things seemed impossible. He knew I needed someone on earth to push me to finish this book. He knew I needed you. Thank you for being that person. Love you, girl!

Exceptional Women

Thank you for trusting me to walk you down the exceptional road. Your patience, kindness, and love inspired me daily to help and guide you on your mission to meet your goals. When I started the Exceptional Health Masterclass I had a vision, but I had no idea of the outcome on the other side. Thank you for letting me be a part of your amazing transformations. I love every one of you.

Jesus Christ my Lord and Savior

As a little girl, I always knew you were with me. You were the one that got me through the night when I was scared as I sang, "Jesus Loves Me." When I learned You died for me and my sins, I didn't think I was good enough. But you put your arms around me and walked down the aisle with me as I sang, "I Have Decided to Follow Jesus." As I grew and wasn't sure what direction to go, you led me as I sang, "Thy Word." When I lost my first baby and couldn't voice how I was feeling. You were there telling me you would take care of her. When I felt like I couldn't handle another day and wanted to run away, You would comfort me and say hold on one more day. As I was writing this book and the fears would come up and stop me from taking the next step, you were there cheering me on. Thank you, Jesus, for not giving up on me. Thank you for loving me unconditionally day after day and bringing people in my life to show me I could love myself unconditionally too.

Cover Design: Shawna Cale
Photo: Sonja Marie Photography

Prologue

Normal.

If I heard that word one more time, I would scream.

I was tired of normal!

I wanted more for me, for my family, my friends, for women around the world.

I was ready to start a rebellion against NORMAL.

If normal is... sickness, fatigue, pain, headaches, depression, arthritis, miscarriages, obesity, diabetes, cancer, anxiety, disease... then

Normal is Highly Overrated.

How did we get here? How did we become a society where being "normal" is the American dream?

Must it take nearly dying to wake up and say, "Normal is not good enough?"

I choose different. I choose exceptional.

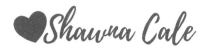

Contents

Introduction

The Road to Health

"Two roads diverged in a wood, and I -
I took the one less traveled by,
and that has made all the difference."
~ Robert Frost

Do you know what road you are traveling?
Where your current pathway is leading you?

Many of us take the path of least resistance, the one the world is following, it often seems to be the right road, it has the bright lights — the shiny billboards — signs at every corner. It has most people saying:

> >FOLLOW ME<<

Do we ever question where that road is going —
the results we will achieve?

What I learned from my first 40 years of life—much like the Israelites' 40-year journey in the wilderness searching for the Promised Land—is the "normal" road leads to dis-ease. It often takes you in circles and just when you think you are getting closer to the results you wish, you find you are just as far away today as you were 10 years ago. It wasn't until I asked questions—to God and to myself—that I understood where the road was going. I needed to exit off the path I was traveling before I found my health at a point of no return—a diagnosis.

We often assume when we get to the place—where we hear—"You've got..." we will stop and choose another road. **But we are habitual beings and our earlier choices, experiences, challenges and even traumas on the way don't just disappear.** It's what we know—it's as if we are on automatic pilot and we wake up finding ourselves back on that road—even when we realize it is the one that brought us where we are today.

This book is two parts and can serve you two ways. Part 1—My story, I share it because I believe so often as women we think everyone else is living the perfect way of life and we are the only ones "broken" and alone.

I want you to recognize you are not alone. Your story—a life of experiences that have led you to where you are today does not define who you are as a person or who God created you to be. On my journey I discovered understanding my story helped me figure out what was blocking my path of holistic health and sharing myself wholly with others. You too can use your story to find your way.

God is a part of my daily life and I share scripture along with scientific research to connect how our spiritual, emotional, and physical health plays a part in the healing process. I believe God is our creator and I give Him the glory for the direction He has set me on and called me to share with you.

Part 2—The Roadmap, I share the formula God gave me to help me choose the road less traveled. These chapters are like a roadmap full of treasures leading you to your "exceptional" life—pointing to a relationship with God and holistic health.

Consider me your friend and personal tour guide. It's my pleasure to walk with you. Together we will experience heartaches, challenges, and adventures as I show you paths, roads, and exits you may take along the way. I will even share my favorite tips and tools to empower you to be the CEO of your own life.

As your tour guide, my mission is to help keep you on track and prevent you from getting lost on the way. Have you had seasons wandering the desert looking for a destination only to see another mirage? There is hope. This quest is not a vacation. It's not short term or even about reaching the dream location by the end. It's life. (The end of your journey is when it's your time to leave this earth.) I say this because I often pick up a book to read, assuming what the author knows will "fix" me and by the end of the book everything will be "perfect." I compare it to planning a dream vacation... where we only picture the best parts—in this dream, we place high expectations on ourselves, on others, and on the destination itself. Life is not perfect and many things in this world we have no control over, we find ourselves disillusioned, discouraged, and disappointed.

What if we figure out how living our dream life may be the actions we take today to live out our purpose tomorrow?

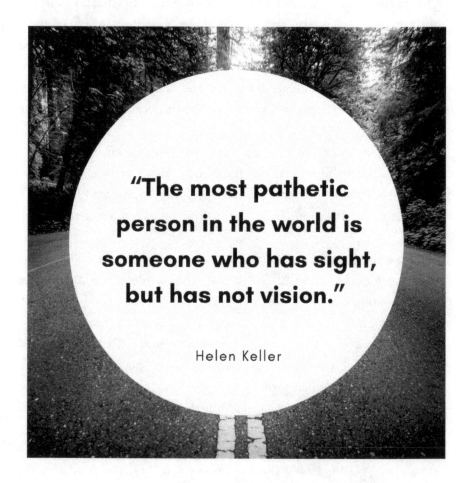

"The most pathetic person in the world is someone who has sight, but has not vision."

Helen Keller

My desire is, as you read, you dream of what's possible for your EXCEPTIONAL life. You realize how this formula directs you to the probable. When you have a "vision," it leads you to hope.

"And the Lord answered me, and said, Write the vision, and make it plain upon tablets, that he may run that readeth it."

HABAKKUK 2:2 (KJV)

It's important to let your imagination dare to dream what you may believe is impossible, and capture the passion that will catapult you to the person you choose to be, living out your purpose.

"Where there is no vision, the people perish: but he that keepeth the law, happy is he."

PROVERBS 29:18 (KJV)

It is not our abilities or our past or current circumstances that limit us. Our vision of what can *be* is what limits us. A vision is not just a picture of what could be; it's a call to become something more...

Are you ready to become more?

Throughout this book, I am going to stop my dialogue and ask you questions. I believe it's important to pause, reflect, and think about the question before moving on. Think of it as the two of us taking a walk and talking. The questions I am asking will help you receive the full benefit of this book—growth. These same questions will be in the journal pages at www.shawnacale.com/book-bonus.

In each chapter, I will give you a challenge, action, and/or exercise to complete that will lead you towards an exceptional life. Of course, it's your choice whether you want to take part, but I have found when I set back and consume nothing changes, I don't change. When I follow through is when I grow. If you skip one, you can always go back and do it later, it just may take you longer to get where you want to be. By the time we finish, you may choose to say *Bye Bye Normal—Hello Exceptional*, like me.

What the Lord has given me has been powerful and has helped me transform beyond what I ever thought was possible. I desire the same for you.

> *"For God has not given us a spirit of fear and timidity, but of power, love, and self-discipline."*
> ### 2 TIMOTHY 1:7 (NLT)

This verse tells us—you and I—we have power. The word for power in this scripture is *dunamis*[1], which is the English word for dynamite. As we travel down the road to health, I have some bonus material that I call TNT (Tips and Tools) to help you blast through spiritual, emotional, and physical blockers as you find faith, love, and self-discipline on your journey.

Whenever you see the TNT icon go to www.shawnacale.com/book-bonus to further guide you through the process. I'll be providing various resources—including journal pages, graphics, questionnaires, lists, assessments, videos, and information to empower you every step of the way. As your friend, I recommend stopping right here and completing the first challenge, and then we can move forward together.

Go to www.shawnacale.com/book-bonus
Printable Journal Pages and Bonus Resources
to Live an Exceptional Life.

CHALLENGE: VISION

1. Pick a quiet place where you can relax with nothing to interrupt you.

2. Let your imagination go—picture yourself having what you have always dreamed of having, doing what you want to do, going to the places you have always wanted to go... picture yourself as the person you were born to be.

3. Begin writing your vision, your dreams, your goals. You can draw pictures, cut out pictures, glue them on your paper, doodle, write a story, or a little of everything. It is up to you; there is no right or wrong way.

PART 1

My Story

Bye Bye Normal

"This is my story, this is my song
Praising my Savior all the day long"
~ Fanny Crosby

I

The Penny

"Trust in the Lord with all your heart and lean not on your
own understanding; in all your ways submit to him,
and he will make your paths straight."
~ Proverbs 3:5-6 (NIV)

Have you ever walked down a path and your eyes come upon a golden object lying in the sun, all bright and shiny, calling your name to pick it up? You find it's a little penny and your thoughts go straight to the poem.

FIND A PENNY, PICK IT UP.
ALL DAY LONG YOU'LL HAVE GOOD LUCK.

You take the penny and place it in your pocket, thinking of all the good it may bring you. I hope this book will be like that penny and bring you good luck along the way, as you read the words that bring my story to you.

My youngest son, Bryce, and I like to play this game in our minivan, where he grabs a stack of pennies from the coin holder and looks at the "heads" side, and tells me the year. My part in the game is storyteller, and for each year he gives me I tell him a short story of something that happened in my life that year, each one a glimpse into the good life I have lived. He loves the game and I love to tell stories. I would love to share with you what I like to call my penny story.

THE HEADS SIDE

"One penny may seem to you a very insignificant thing,
but it is the small seed from which fortunes spring."
~ Orison Swett Marden

1970–It was the year I was born, right around Thanksgiving to a young woman who loved me very much. It's the reason Thanksgiving is my favorite holiday; it's a time to celebrate and show gratitude to those we love. My mom is someone I will always be thankful for and whom I love very much.

1971–I grew up in a typical American home with Mom, Dad, and my little brother, who was born when I was just a little over a year old. I loved my little brother, and we were the best of friends. In the eyes of the world, I am sure we looked like the perfect American family. We even have pictures to prove it.

1973–I smile. That was the year my parents bought a brand-new house, and I grew up on a street with a cul-de-sac and a gigantic climbing tree across the way. We spent years riding our tricycles and Big Wheel down the driveway and, as we got older, our bikes all over the street and through the neighborhood. I had lots of friends and we would play all day at one another's houses. It was the best of times and we were happy.

1975–Oh, the fun our family had as we spent weekends at the lake during the summer. We started out camping in a tent and then moving up to a camper on the back of our baby blue pickup truck. I loved riding in the front of our boat with my long blonde hair flying as I sang songs in the wind. We would swim and ride on our zip sled and later learn to water ski. I remember at the campgrounds people thinking my brother and I were twins and we would play along with that idea. We found people loved to give gifts to twins. We had so much fun and joy in our lives.

1976–I remember being so excited to start kindergarten. One particular day the summer before I started school, my parents picked me up from daycare for a special trip to downtown Oklahoma City. We went to the tallest building I had ever seen. It was something we had to do before I could start school, and it was the most wonderful day ever. I loved everything about school! Books, recess, and playing with Play-Doh were my three favorite things, but the highlight of my day was the reading circle where I learned to read from the *Dick and Jane* books. Learning to read made me feel confident in myself. My dad would read to me at night or I would read to him. My mom also stayed home that year and was the classroom mom. She taught me how to cook and I would play house with my wooden kitchen set and cook for my baby dolls. I couldn't wait to be a mom one day.

1977–That was the year we bought my favorite dress for Easter. It was a long pink dress with a little bell on the bottom that would ring when I would walk. I loved spending the holidays with the family and seeing my grandparents, my aunts, uncles, and cousins. All the wonderful food, too. My grandma made the best strawberry shortcake and one of my aunts made the best fudge, my mom would bring the candied yams with the melted marshmallows to all the holiday gatherings, I remember lots of laughter and delightful times as we celebrated. I also loved riding the church bus on Sundays. It was my favorite day of the week. Saturday night after my bath, mom would roll my hair with pink foam curlers while we watched *Little House on the Prairie* as a family. The next morning, I would wake up early to put on my favorite dress—the pink one as often as I could. I loved dresses and feeling like a princess.

1978–Mrs. Kidwell, my favorite teacher ever. She was so funny, and she was always writing poems and putting them on the chalkboard for us to write in cursive. She wrote one about me and my best friend: I was spaghetti head because of my long straight blonde hair and she was macaroni because her last name was Roney. We laughed all day, maybe all year long about our special poem. Maybe it was Mrs. Kidwell who taught me the penny rhyme; I know she sparked my love for poetry. We had so many adventures in that class... like the time the skunks lived under our classroom in the annex... or how she would teach an entire math lesson by talking into the fan because we didn't have an air conditioner. She would even let us bring the record player as close to the door that led outside so we could have dance parties during recess. Still, to this day, second grade was my favorite year ever!

1979–That was the year we went on our first trip to Six Flags Over Texas. There was a huge roller coaster called the *Shock Wave*, and everyone wanted to ride it except me. It was big and had two loops. I'm sure my knees were knocking and my stomach was hurting because I just knew if I rode it I would die. Guess what? I was just as afraid to wait all by myself at the bottom while everyone else rode the roller coaster. I found the courage to get on, and it was the most exhilarating feeling I had ever experienced... so much fear and excitement all rolled into one. By the time the ride was over, I loved roller coasters and was ready for any new adventure.

1980–That was the year of change. At the end of 1979, during Christmas break, we moved across the United States to Virginia for my dad's job. I was excited about moving to a far-off place and meeting new people and having a two-story house. We spent much of the year visiting a quaint town called Occoquan, taking my first trip to the ocean, and visiting Washington, D.C. I loved it all, but one of my favorite memories was buying a book at the Smithsonian Institution called *Women Pioneers of Science*.[1] I told everyone that when I grew up, I would be a doctor and help people like the women in the book.

I just shared with you a decade's worth of penny memories. These are the stories I tell my children and the rest of the world. My life filled with good luck, just like that penny in my pocket.

TWO SIDES

"Why can't I remember that not once have I ever seen a coin,
whether grimy copper or bright gold, that had but one side."
~ Andrew Levkoff

We often forget that every penny has two sides. I am sure if a penny could talk it would have a lot to say. The "heads" would tell one beautiful story after another of good luck it had brought to the people it touched through the years. It would tell us all the wonderful places it had been, with whom, and what it had seen and done—the worth it had contributed to this world.

But what about the "tails" side? It may not have a year engraved on it, but I am sure it would share as many if not more stories... All the bad luck it had experienced falling to the ground, person after person passing it by. The "tails" would tell of becoming lost and falling deep into a drain after being kicked over and over in the dirt, and how it felt like a failure, of not being enough, being left behind, and just wanting someone, anyone, to want it enough to pick it up and put it in a safe pocket with the other pennies.

You may relate to what I like to call my "heads" stories, but you may have also thought, "I wish I had been as lucky as she." Many people have said to me: "You are so lucky." And though I have been blessed, and I love sharing all my wonderful experiences, there are two sides to every penny and my story is no different.

THE TAILS SIDE

"Do not pick up a tails up penny."
~ Unknown

My husband and I were watching a show on TV, and my heart ached. Not like heartburn, or stabbing pain, but a deep, deep, down-to-the-soul kind of ache. It's the ache when someone has something removed, leaving a black hole that is so far down that it is unreachable. The pain almost too much to bear. It's a pain that is most often felt with sadness and grief.

I am not sure why the show elicited this pain. Maybe empathy for the mom in the story, but the heartache is an ache I have not felt so deeply for almost ten years. That night started my journey of telling my story and writing this book, but it was not the first time I felt this ache, and my guess is it will not be the last.

I planned to go to bed and go to sleep. But, as I lay there with this pain in my heart, all I could think about is writing these next words for anyone who has felt this same ache or will one day go through something that leaves a hole they don't know how to fill.

I wish I could sit down in front of every woman and share my story. My whole story. Not because my story is special, exciting, or so different from most. It's because when we share stories—the real, raw stories, the ones so many of us are afraid to share—it connects us. It allows us to see we are not alone. What we are going through is part of our journey here on earth and we don't have to suffer, live in fear, confusion, alone. We can lean on one another, share what we have gone through, and know that we are safe, free of judgment, and free to be who God has made us to be.

Why is it that our circumstances often write the story we keep inside, define our self-worth, and take the joy out of our journey?

Is that why my heart ached while I watched this show? Seeing this woman, this mom with a broken heart who had no control over those around her and nothing she could do to "fix" the problem.

There is no going back; there is only learning from our past, choosing to move forward. No matter how hard the future looks and no matter how much it hurts, the present is where we live and the future is only our dream of tomorrow.

I write. The pain lessens. That's how life is, with time, new seasons, the pain changes, we change. Growth is difficult, but stagnation—being stuck—is not living, it's only surviving.

As I share the other side of my story—the "tails" side—I hope you get to know me a little better than most.

THE OTHER SIDE

"There is always the other side."
~ Jean Rhys

1970–When I was born, it was just my mom and me; no husband and no father. Only 16 percent of women were unwed mothers. It wasn't the "norm." I know it must not have been an easy choice to keep a baby at such a young age. We lived with my grandma in a trailer behind her purple bar on a highway outside of town—what many would call "the other side of the tracks."

1971–My mom got married and had my little brother. I was now a big girl and felt the expectations to be a big helper. It's hard to admit, but I was jealous of my little brother and, although I loved him, I also resented him.

1973–My maternal grandmother was murdered. My mom was young, and I can only imagine how traumatic it would be to lose your mother at such a young age. Since I was only a few years old, I remember little about my grandma. I can see her hands and her feet in my memories, but not her face. I so want to remember her face and I often will place the photo I have seen of her into my memories, but it's just a photograph.

My grandma owned a bar and I can still remember the door, the counter, the pool table with a light above it, but my eyes always take me back to the chip clip on the wall as I hear my grandma ask me, "Which one do you want?" Seeing her hand go over the choices—Ruffles, Fritos... stopping at the Cheetos as I ask for them. She hands me the chips and my gaze moves down to the bag in my hands... it's then that I see her funny little silver slippers with pointed-up toes. But it's her face I wish I could remember. It's her touch I long for, but all I can see are those chips.

Soon after the funeral, our typical American family broke apart: Mom and Dad got divorced and my brother and I spent weekends between parents. I don't have a lot of memories during that time, only feelings of sadness, and it being an unknown, unsafe, and unstable time. Maybe when my grandma died or my dad (that's what I called him) left is when I felt that first deep ache within my heart.

My mom worked, so my brother and I went to daycare. I always wanted my mom to stay at home with us. A few of the neighbor moms were home during the day, and I had aunts that were too. Being so young, I didn't understand why she worked. I remember one rainy morning after being dropped off at daycare, running and crying to the window, watching my mom get back into her car and leave. I wanted my mom, and I can still feel the crushing pain in my heart. I knew she loved me; I knew she had to go, but I wanted her to stay and take me home. I wanted her to take the pain away.

1976–Mom and Dad remarried, and my dad adopted me. The "heads" story I told about going to the tall building in Oklahoma City happened that day. I thought all kids did this before they went to kindergarten. It's hard for a small child to understand adoption, but to me, it felt like a special, happy day. I went alone into this room with dark walls and a man sitting behind an enormous desk to answer some questions. I remember him telling me I had pretty blue eyes. That was something I heard often, and I had my standard reply: "Thank you, I got them from my daddy." The judge replied, "You know your dad?" At this point, I thought judges were stupid, or kindergarten would be easy. I was a spunky little five-year-old and replied with an eye roll and a "yes" as I pointed to my mom and dad, who was standing at the door. He then asked the second most stupid question I had ever heard. "Do you love your dad?" Again, my answer was "yes" and then I remember everyone smiling and papers being signed.

THE DARK SIDE

"My glorious dark side, Listen to me now, Let me find light..."
~ Poojitha Kankatala

As I tell this side of the story and share my feelings, it's hard to see that there is much difference between the heads and the tails—just a few more details that most leave out. However, many people believe that the "tails" side of the penny is the dark, evil side. There was also a dark side of my childhood: The side I hid and where anger grew and tried to define who I was as a person.

I was molested by not just one man, but three: my Grandpa (adopted dad's father), my friend's dad (our neighbor across the street), and a babysitter's teenage son.

I could just stop right here. Trust has been a big issue for me. It's hard enough to trust those I love. We need trust to connect with others. Trust may be an issue for you, too. Maybe you were hurt or betrayed and the only way you know how to protect yourself is to keep people at a distance. That's where I have lived for years—building a wall around my heart to protect myself. That's what you do when you don't feel safe to be you, to be in your own body, to live in this world. It's where I feel most comfortable, even today. But here is where I choose to get vulnerable with you.

Part of me wants to turn the penny back over to the good side and move on, but as I said, when we share our stories—the real, raw stories that many of us are afraid to share—we become connected. On the "heads" side of the penny are the words, "In God We Trust." I am writing this book—I am doing the hard things by putting my trust in God so we can find healing. If I continue to hide behind the circumstances that happened in my life, the experiences that formed my beliefs, then I let those circumstances dictate my story. I choose to grow and learn from those times and I hope as I share my feelings, my healing, you can learn through me.

One thing I have learned through writing my story is finding the value in my painful life experiences. I never wanted to play a victim or let my past affect my present or my future. I would much rather ignore the past and dream of the future. But many women today feel alone, hurt, confused, overwhelmed, misunderstood, worn-out, and weighed down by past life experiences. I too was one of those women.

Limiting beliefs are built on stories from a child's viewpoint that tell us we are not good enough, broken, not worthy.[2] These beliefs bring up thoughts we play in our heads, wondering if things had been different, would we be different? The emotions created we work so hard to bury, only to find our energy drained without even knowing or understanding why.

When we find meaning and purpose even in the bad, hurtful experiences are when we can heal our soul and find joy in the journey. I don't want to just journey through life; I want joy in my journey. How about you? Are you tired of just surviving or moving through life as if on a conveyor belt where you have no say where you go? I know I am. So here I go, sharing my painful life experiences to bring value to those experiences. I am flipping the penny over to the "tails" side and guess what it says? *e pluribus unum.* What does that funny Latin phrase mean? "Out of many, one." This phrase, to me, means that each of us has our own stories, different from one another, not better or worse, just different, but when we share our stories, we become one. The penny poem says nothing about the "tails" side being bad luck.

FIND A PENNY,
PICK IT UP,
ALL THE DAY,
YOU'LL HAVE GOOD LUCK
GIVE IT TO A FAITHFUL FRIEND,
THEN YOUR LUCK WILL NEVER END!

 I am giving YOU, my faithful friend, a penny as a reminder YOU are not alone.

THE OLD RUSTY PENNY

"A bad penny always turns up."
- Unknown

Grandpa always told me I was special, and all the sweet things little girls like to hear. He always told me how pretty I was when I would wear a dress. He picked me to sit on his lap while all the other kids played. He would give me a half-dollar and tell the older cousins to take us younger ones to the Dairy Boy for ice cream. I loved ice cream. The other kids would get enough money for an ice cream cone, but I always had enough for my favorite—a maraschino cherry sundae. I was special. I felt special. I felt loved.

One day when we got home from my grandparent's house I had to pee, and it burned. I told my mom, and she asked a few questions. I told her the truth: "Maybe because of Grandpa's hands." I could tell from her expression that what I was telling her was bad. I am not sure how long it had been going on, but I knew that Grandpa had been making me feel special for a long time. I remember Mom and Dad screaming and yelling in the other room as I sat there all alone on the toilet.

Grandpa wasn't the only one who loved me and made me feel special. There was a neighbor across the street. I figured out on my own what he was doing must be bad, too. I was too scared to tell my mom or anyone else about him. My mom told me to let no one touch me there again. I felt like I was a bad little girl, even though I was told it wasn't my fault and Grandpa should have never touched me there. The problem was—I liked how it made me feel, and it made me think I must be bad, too.

We didn't visit my grandparents for what seemed like forever; I am not sure how long, just a year or several years, but I know we missed Christmas and Easter, two of my favorite times of the year.

As an adult, I believe that my parents did what was best. I had good parents doing all they knew to do. I didn't know these men in my life groomed me—they gained my trust, filled my needs of attention, gift-giving, and created a powerful bond, one that kept me silent for way too long.

Here is where I get vulnerable, feelings I just don't share with others. Tell someone you have been molested and you're the innocent kid. But I did not grow up feeling innocent. I felt by telling the truth; I was being punished. I no longer saw my family. As if someone whom I loved, who loved me and made me feel special, was taken from me. I didn't want to feel that way; I hated myself for feeling the way I did.

**Have you ever thought your "feelings" were wrong?
Have you ever let someone hurt you because the
alternative of being alone felt even worse?**

THE DIRTY PENNY

"The first part in healing is shattering the silence."
~ Erin Merryn

I still had the situation with the neighbor's dad, and I didn't want play-time with my friends taken from me, too. I was still special in his eyes, but now I felt like I was playing a part in the evil that I now knew existed. I was no longer the innocent child not knowing any better. I compare it to how Adam and Eve felt the day they realized they were naked and hid from God. Now that I knew it was bad, I felt guilty every time, but I wanted to go—I wanted to feel loved, I wanted to feel special. Yet, I felt dirty and yucky and awful at the same time.

The spiritual fight within me was strong—as if I was two different people: the sweet, pretty little girl that everyone saw on the outside and the bad, ugly little girl that I knew lived inside. I have learned a lot about myself as an adult, and one thing I have learned is that I see everything through the lens of right and wrong, good and bad. I became a liar and let my circumstances tell me who I was as a person. I was bad, but I couldn't let anyone know that I was bad, so I had to be right.

THE LIAR PENNY

"Silence is a protective coating over pain."
~ E. Lockart

My brother and I went to a babysitter who had a teenage son. I didn't like to take naps; I just wanted to read. I thought I was too old and too mature to take naps. I was maybe 7 or 8 years old. I think being molested makes a little girl grow up faster. The babysitter would turn off all the lights, which made reading very difficult, and I would complain. Her son had a marvelous idea—I could read in his room. His mom agreed. By this time, I could feel the signs. I knew what he was thinking, and I felt the evil within. I wanted to just say "no." I knew that was the right thing to do. What good girls would do. But the thought of someone new wanting me felt good too, and I wanted to read. His room was off-limits for the other kids, I would be the special one. Just thinking back to that time makes my stomach hurt. My stomach hurt a lot as a child. Even though I knew it was wrong and I knew what would happen, I would go to his room for naptime every day. Again, the sweet, innocent girl was not so sweet and innocent, and I lived in fear that someone would find out.

Around the same time, a teenage girl would come over and babysit my brother and me on the weekends. She would bring cigarettes. I wanted to be a teenager like her so I would show her pornographic magazines that I had found in a drawer, and she would let me smoke a cigarette in the bathroom while taking a bath as we looked at porn—one more thing to hide and lie to my parents about. Lying was becoming second nature. I felt everything about my life was a lie.

> "Lying was becoming second nature. I felt everything about my life was a lie."

THE SPINNING PENNY

"I think there is a danger... of this spinning out of control."
~ Richard Dicker

Ever feel like your life is spinning out of control? That's how I was feeling during this time. One day at school a girl in my class told me that her real parents didn't love her, and they gave her away to these people who adopted her. I remembered the word *adoption* from my happy day at the high rise in Oklahoma City. Was that the problem? Was I adopted? Did my real parents not love me, so they gave me away? Is that why I was bad?

I asked my mom about it. She explained that she was my real mother and that my dad adopted me. I asked questions about my actual dad, but she didn't say much, just that he didn't want her or me. I played it off as "I was special." I reasoned that Dad paid for me because he loved me so much, but inside I felt unwanted, alone, and hurt.

I remember hating my life so much by the summer after second grade I packed up my Big Mac Attack backpack and I was going to run away. I thought I was old enough to take care of myself and even find a job and live on my own. I know it sounds ridiculous, but I remember it like it was yesterday, and everything in me thought I could do it. Luckily, my mom stopped me. She loved me and she made sure I knew it. I didn't feel that I deserved her love. I was a terrible, evil little girl living inside a body that seemed to only get me in trouble.

I thought if I couldn't run away, I would kill myself. I had learned at school you should never put a plastic bag over your face or you could suffocate and die. I went searching for plastic and all I found was a plastic sandwich bag. I put it over my face—breathed in and out—nothing. I wasn't dying. I remember lying under my bed crying, wanting the pain inside to stop. My heart ached, and I felt so alone, and I knew that I could tell no one my secrets. If they knew the real me, they would hate me and see me for who I was—a bad girl.

THE TURNING PENNY

"That was the turning point."
~ Anthony Parham

We moved to Virginia when I was 9. I am sure it was God's way of protecting me from the men in my life and from myself. It was a hard move for me because I had lots of friends at school and it was the one place that I felt safe and good about myself. It was also hard because I no longer could spend time at the neighbor's house and that's where I felt most special.

I felt so alone in Virginia. Things were different, people were different. I was the same. I thought this was a new beginning—a chance for me to be a good girl, yet; I remember lying in bed wondering what neighbor would want me and what I would do if he tried anything. It was like I was fighting myself on what was right and what I wanted or didn't want to happen. Nothing happened. Then I found out we were moving back to Oklahoma. I was so excited. I would see my friends again, I would be back in my house, my neighborhood.

While we were gone, a lot changed. My best friend moved and the neighbor friend with the father who molested me was moving too. Part of me was glad, but that didn't stop me from going to their new house when given the opportunity. I was older now; I thought chances were good that nothing would happen. I would just make sure to not be alone with him. When he picked up me and my brother in his truck, he made me sit next to him. With his hand down my pants on the lengthy drive to his house, I knew nothing had changed. I had not changed.

That weekend was the last time he ever molested me. I was 10 years old, and I decided when I went home that weekend that I would never, ever let a man make me feel dirty again. I would take control of my life and nobody would ever hurt me.

As I look back, I am very proud of myself for making grown-up decisions at an early age, but I built up beliefs that were not true. I thought love was the sexual feelings that I felt. I thought those feelings were bad.

So, when I decided to no longer allow men to touch me, I also decided I didn't want to feel loved, or be special.

THE LOST PENNY

"I once was lost but now am found."
~ John Newton

I grew up riding a church bus to Sunday School. I loved singing songs, playing games, and learning about Jesus. I don't remember a time not believing in God. He was my safe place. Though I didn't understand what it meant to have a relationship with Him, or about Jesus dying for my sins, or even what sin was, I understood He was good, and the devil was bad. I knew singing *Jesus Loves Me* at night when I felt the evil within boiling up would allow me to sleep. I knew God was the one who saved me from running away and trying to end my life. The only way I can explain it "I just knew."

When we returned from Virginia, we started going to church as a family, or at least my mom, brother, and I went most Sundays. I remember hearing a message about everyone having skeletons in their closet—the secret sins people keep from others but that God knew about. I enjoyed the message because I now felt I was not alone—others had secrets, too. But I didn't like the thought of a good God or others knowing my terrible sins.

As the weeks went by my mom gave her life to Christ by saying a prayer that she wanted Him as her Lord and Savior. I wasn't ready. How could a wonderful God love me? Maybe if I stayed good a while longer God could forgive me, but not yet. I had only recently decided to "not" let anyone touch me.

As I sat in the pew at church one Sunday we sang, *I Have Decided to Follow Jesus* and I experienced God. It was as if a warm blanket of protection wrapped itself all around me while I was singing. I felt loved; I felt special in a beautiful way, not the way the men in my life had made me feel special. At that moment I knew I wanted to feel that way forever: safe, loved, wanted. I walked to the front of the church and gave my life to Christ. I prayed a simple prayer, and I asked Him into my heart. When I tell others that on March 8, 1981, when I was 10 years old, I made the most life-changing decision, I'm almost certain they are thinking I was too young to make that kind of decision or that I didn't understand what it was like to have my sins forgiven. I understood. I may have been only 10, but that was a day of freedom for me.

In the Bible, there is a story that Jesus tells in Luke Chapter 15 about a lost coin that was found. I always picture that coin like a penny, safe and protected in God's hands, not alone or forgotten. No longer was I lost—I was found.

THE LOST COIN

"Or suppose a woman has ten silver coins and loses one. Doesn't she light a lamp, sweep the house and search carefully until she finds it? And when she finds it, she calls her friends and neighbors together and says, 'Rejoice with me; I have found my lost coin.' In the same way, I tell you, there is rejoicing in the presence of the angels of God over one sinner who repents."
LUKE 15:8-10 (NIV)

Amazing Grace

Amazing Grace, how sweet the sound,
That saved a wretch like me.
I once was lost but now am found,
Was blind, but now I see.

T' was Grace that taught my heart to fear.
And Grace, my fears relieved.
How precious did that Grace appear
The hour I first believed.

Through many dangers, toils and snares
I have already come;
'Tis Grace that brought me safe thus far
and Grace will lead me home.

The Lord has promised good to me.
His word my hope secures.
He will my shield and portion be,
As long as life endures.

Yea, when this flesh and heart shall fail,
And mortal life shall cease,
I shall possess within the veil,
A life of joy and peace.

When we've been there ten thousand years
Bright shining as the sun.
We've no less days to sing God's praise
Than when we've first begun.

by John Newton

THE NEW PENNY

"Take life one day at a time because every day
is a different day with new challenges."
~ Penny Streeter

I wish I could say that becoming a Christian changed my life into this beautiful, wonderful, perfect thing. It did not. I was reborn; I was new, and I had an incredible strength from the Lord that I did not have before. I am not sure I would have made it through my teenage years without God. It was difficult enough with Him. God did not promise a perfect life on earth, He promised He would always be there for me and He has always been faithful.

> *"So do not fear, for I am with you; do not be dismayed, for I am your God. I will strengthen you and help you; I will uphold you with my righteous right hand."*
> ISAIAH 41:10 (NIV)

In our first years of life, we create beliefs. The wonderful experiences I shared created beliefs. The terrible experiences I shared created beliefs. Both make up who we are and what we think about ourselves and others. Looking deep into your own personal story is not always easy, but I found understanding my stories helped me better understand what I was feeling like as a child and why I've felt the way I've felt throughout my life. What I have learned on my journey to spiritual, emotional, and physical health is that those beliefs affect every part of our life.

You are both sides of the penny. Every penny has the same worth assigned to it, no matter if it lands on its "heads" or its "tails", if it's spinning, rusty, dirty, or even brand new. I want you to know that your circumstances, your beliefs, your emotions, your feelings, your actions, your results do not determine your worth. God paid the same price for every one of us. He sent his Son to die for every person, no matter what they have done or not done. The truth is: You are worthy, you are good enough, you are special, you are unconditionally loved—and so am I.

My journey has been letting the little girl inside me believe this as much as she believes it for other women. My desire is to give you the Tips and Tools (power) to move from limiting beliefs created from your view-point, your experiences, and your feelings into empowering beliefs that take you from "normal" to exceptional.

Go to www.shawnacale.com/book-bonus
Printable Journal Pages and Bonus Resources
to Live an Exceptional Life.

CHALLENGE: PENNY GAME

1. Pick a quiet place where you can relax with nothing to interrupt and journal your childhood story. You will use your stories as we move forward to find your way to healing.

2. Print off the journal pages or take out a piece of paper and write "Heads" at the top. Start writing the memories of your childhood you share with others, the good, life-changing times. They don't have to be complete sentences; they can just be pieces of memories. If you remember years, ages, or grades, write that next to them. This is just for you and need not be perfect.

3. Now start a new piece of paper or flip the paper over to the other side and write "Tails" at the top. Spend a little time on the things you may recall as bad, sad, or that you pretend never happened. You don't have to go into deep detail; just write them down to get them out of your head and onto paper. You don't have to share this side with anyone unless you choose to.

2

The Roller Coaster

Consider it pure joy, my brothers and sisters,
whenever you face trials of many kinds.
~ James 1:2 (NIV)

I built a relationship with God as the world around me seemed to crumble. My parents divorced again, and my brother moved in with my dad after he remarried. It seemed like me and my mom against the world, but God held us in His hands and kept us safe. The stories about that period would fill another book, and maybe one day I will write that one because the lessons I learned from those years are priceless.

School, the one thing that stayed consistent in my life from kindergarten until 9th grade, kept me going. I loved school. I loved learning. I loved escaping into books and forgetting my life while reading about the adventures of others.

I survived the best way I knew how—I took every feeling, every emotion, and stuffed it down as far as it would go—straight into my gut. I started menstruating the first day of 7th grade and had an appendectomy several months later. It would be the start of a quarter of a century of emotional symptoms that included irritability, mood changes, anxiety, depression, and physical symptoms such as abdominal and back pain, acne, breast tenderness, bloating, and feeling drained.

My stomach hurt a lot in Junior High—it felt like that first drop on a roller coaster when you yell and lose your stomach. I didn't understand why it hurt all the time. Now, looking back, I recognize it was stress. All I knew was that my parents were going through a divorce and family life was not fun. I hate to admit it, but I lived on Snickers and Sprite for lunch, and whatever my mom and I would come up with for dinner. I began an unhealthy connection to food to comfort the girl who was hurting spiritually, emotionally, and physically and was too scared to let anyone know she needed help.

Has food, particularly sweet treats, ever comforted you?

Some people turn to drugs, alcohol, and other destructive addictions. I found happiness in a candy bar and a soda pop. Innocent enough, right?

I thought by hiding my feelings and turning to what made me feel good—ice cream and other sweet treats—I could get through the days until I became an adult and lived my own life. I believed as an adult I could control my own circumstances. My dream was to live the "normal" American life because my past seemed anything but. I remember telling one of my closest friends about being molested, and I still remember the look on her face. I did not want her sympathy. I didn't think I deserved her sympathy. I figured that everything that happened was my fault. I let them do what they did. Anytime an emotion regarding my childhood surfaced, I pushed it down even further. I would protect myself from harm by not feeling anything at all. I would keep my secret from the world. I would not be the victim.

Note: The Subheadings are names of actual roller coasters around the world.

TRANSITION - RISE OF THE RESISTANCE

"Resistance to change is always the biggest obstacle."
~ Chris Paine

Have you ever wanted something so much, but resisted it at the same time? I wanted to be "normal" like all the other girls. But it didn't seem like that was my lot in life. My parents were divorced and though that was the "norm" for my family (most of my aunts and uncles had been married and divorced) that was not the "norm" of my closest friends. I enjoyed hanging out with my friends and their families to see what a marriage and family could look like. I was the "good girl" at school and resisted "normal" teenage fun. Not necessarily a bad thing, but always felt outside of the loop.

I found peace from the angst of my hormonal/emotional roller coaster with the use of ibuprofen, time spent in the library with a book, or hidden away in my room safe from the world—or the world safe from me. I learned how to resist the world by closing myself off. Not necessarily a good thing.

In ninth grade, my mom and I moved back to the city after living in a small town for five years. Coming back to my old house, my old neighborhood and a new high school in Oklahoma City was hard—the good memories, the bad memories, all rolled into one. Drugs were the "norm" for many of these kids, and so many of them were trying to figure out their sexual orientation. I made it through one semester, but I didn't know if I could resist all the evil around me for another year. It was so strong, and I could feel the pull to return to what *Star Wars* fans would call "the dark side." Thoughts of running away and suicide rose inside again but would be quickly replaced by the thoughts of how much God loved me. I knew I had to stay in the church and stay strong for both me and my mom. It was tiring.

The following year I resisted going to the school in our district. By God's grace, I moved in with one of my best friends and her family so I could return to the school and people that were my anchor. It was a time of both rest and trust that God would protect my mom without me being there all the time. I was immersed inside a family that showed unconditional love for one another and gave me hope that I too could one day have a family that stayed together.

My mom the following year moved us into an apartment across the street from the school. Life mostly was good. I liked boys, and I wanted a boyfriend, but how I felt about myself and males made dating a guy in high school difficult. I liked a lot of guys, but I kept them at arm's length. When one would start liking me it didn't take long for me to find something wrong with him and move on to "liking" the next guy. The longest I dated a guy was two weeks. As soon as he told me he loved me it was time to say goodbye. I knew what he wanted, and he wasn't getting it from me—I would resist. I would break the family curse—I would *not* be a teenage mom.

While finding my place in the world, I learned to hide what I did not want people to see and act "normal." Normal for me included acting like the "good, perfect girl." I was the teacher's pet, an excellent student, the girl anyone could tell their problems to, the loyal friend, and the daughter who would do no wrong. Normal also included acne, headaches, joint pain, terrible cramping, and excessive bleeding. I assumed I was doing a good job of being a "normal" teenager while resisting the "normal" negative teenage behaviors. Again, I found this exhausting and couldn't wait to grow up and just be "me."

Determined to go to college and become whoever I wanted to be, I again found that the struggle was real. My step-mom at the time told me I needed to go find myself and that she and my dad would not help me go to college. I didn't feel lost—nor did I feel I needed to find myself. I didn't want their help or anyone's help. I wanted to do it on my own. I knew what I wanted, and I wanted to be a physical therapist. Determined to prove to her and anyone else who tried to get in my way—I would succeed.

I went to the University of Oklahoma alone. All my friends were going to other places, and I was ready for a new start, new friends, a new life. I had this confidence and courage that only God could have given me as I followed His lead. It was difficult; it was scary, lonely, but also exciting, and full of possibilities—a dream-filled future.

I picked out my husband on the first day of my freshman year in Zoology class. I know that may sound funny, but it's true. I had met a girl that asked me if I had a boyfriend and I said no, but I picked out 3 guys in the class that I thought would make the perfect boyfriend. The first one became my husband. The second became a good friend who later was kicked out of school for stealing radios out of cars, and the third sang to me at a dueling piano bar at my bachelorette party.

I met my husband, Kevin, at the first college party I agreed to go to after resisting for several months. It was there I spoke to him and we learned all that we had in common—career, people, even our middle names. I dreamed of this boy one day becoming my husband. It would be several months before we talked again and began dating. It's a love story I know only God could have orchestrated, He knew Kevin was the only one for me.

Physical therapy was a career that many people in the early 1990s competed for, and my chances were slim. However, I would not let my advisor, other teachers, or physical therapists tell me that my dream could not come true. I was persistent and maybe a little "lucky" and grabbed one of the 66 slots that hundreds applied for in 1991 at the University of Oklahoma Health and Sciences Center.

As my relationship grew with Kevin and I trusted him more than any other guy in my life and shared with him my past, I still kept the little girl inside—the one with all the secrets about how she felt about herself—locked up. At least that is what I thought. As part of our pre-marriage counseling, our pastor gave us some tests, which, according to him, showed that I was very hostile. The tests showed what was going on inside of me. I didn't even have a clue what was going on inside of me. I kept it pushed down and hidden, even from myself, but now he told me I would need to let it go.

**Has anyone ever told you to let go
of your feelings and your emotions?**

**Have you ever thought there is no way I can let go
of what I have hidden for so long?**

I realized right then I needed to do a better job at hiding the real
me—the hurt, angry, unworthy little girl who felt so alone. The Rise of
the Resistance would continue to live on.

MARRIAGE - MAGIC MOUNTAIN

*"Marriage is a lot like a roller coaster. You have extreme highs and you can
have some pretty extreme lows, but the ride is worth it."*
~ Teresa Collins

I was young. He was young. We were in love. We were ready to begin
our magical life together. I chose marriage knowing it would be difficult
and assumed with that expectation I wouldn't be disappointed. I figured with determination and the belief of no matter how hard it gets,
I will climb the mountain and I will not give up. My marriage would
make it.

Stress can bring out the "bad" side of anyone and let me tell you
it often reared its ugly head in my marriage. That time of the month
would roll around and my behavior was not pretty. Being on birth control made it even worse—like the bride of Frankenstein.

Because I had trust issues and was hurt by men in my life, I often
kept my husband at a distance. Afraid that if he saw the "real" me, he
wouldn't love me. I asked myself often in the beginning and throughout
our life together, *Can he possibly love me?* I feared if I let him in too deep,
and he left me, it would break my heart. Resisting that deep connection
and keeping him at a distance I presumed would protect my heart from
the pain, I watched my mom and other women in my life go through.

I am a perfectionist—any personality test I take proves it. I wanted
to be the perfect wife, keep the perfect home, fix the perfect meals...

For many years I thought if I just did everything perfectly, it would
be enough. I would be enough. I would have the best life ever. Trust me,

I tried. But things out of my control always seemed to affect my feelings about myself and my life. I did my best, but always felt less than and not enough. My husband deserved more. I needed to love him better. How that looked from the outside was me making him feel worse about himself by criticizing and disrespecting him. If *he* felt less than, then I didn't have to feel so bad about myself. Our marriage made it through both of us graduating college and starting our first full time, grown-up jobs, buying new cars, a new home, everything I had dreamed of except...

MOTHERHOOD - THE HURRICANE

*"To describe my mother would be to write about a
hurricane in its perfect power.
Or the climbing falling colors of a rainbow."*
~ Maya Angelou

My greatest goal in life was to be a mom. I even decided in high school to not pursue being a doctor, my childhood career of choice, when I learned how much time and money it would cost. I couldn't figure out how I could be a stay-at-home mom and a doctor. So, I pursued physical therapy because I wanted babies more.

I'm not sure why I wanted to be a mom so much. I always loved babies. I had several baby dolls growing up and dreamed of them coming alive at night for me to take care of them. I even dreamed that one day someone would leave their baby on my doorstep and ask me to be its mom. I shared with you I picked out my husband in a room full of zoology students. I will admit it was because I thought we would make beautiful babies (I was right).

In 1995, when I found out I would be a mom—my heart was full. During the pregnancy and the first 6 months after his birth, my hormones were on my side for the first time since seventh grade. I loved being a mom. I felt great, relaxed, loving, happy. I wish I could find all the words of how I felt about this little human being that we named

Ryan. He was everything I had ever wanted, and I was determined to be the best mom. Until...

The loop on the hormonal/emotional roller coaster became a non-stop nightmare. I had this desire of being home with my son all the time, yet I felt I needed to help my husband and work to pay the bills. There was also this deep-down belief that one day he could leave me, and I needed to support myself and my son. There was this fight within me and I didn't know what to do, or who I was to be. It scared me; I was lonely, and I didn't know who to confide in—I wanted to be the perfect mom, the perfect wife. The one who had it all together—life all figured out. As time went on, it only got harder. Marriage was difficult. Being a mom was difficult. I learned I did not have control over my child and his behavior, or even the ability to control my own emotions during his outbursts. Toddler, anyone?

I did not like who I was becoming as a mom, wife, woman. It seemed easier to go to work, treat patients than to be the mom I had always dreamed of being. I kept searching for the perfection just around the corner, but never close enough to grasp. There were fulfilling days of love, play, and laughter—more happy than sad—but the feeling inside of me most of the time was not the joy I was seeking. Instead, a raging storm was brewing, and I was waiting for the promise of a rainbow. I loved God; I followed Jesus. Why was I not content?

I had this vision of what my perfect life should look like, and when I reached it I felt overwhelmed and disconnected from those, I loved most. I knew I had everything I ever dreamed of and still felt empty inside. Was I broken? Did I need someone to "fix" me? As a perfectionist, all I knew to do was work harder at being perfect. It was tiring; it was impossible, but it was my only hope.

Have you ever felt broken?
Searching for someone to "fix" you?

MORE BABIES - RAINBOW CHASER

"Everybody wants happiness. Nobody wants pain.
But you can't have a rainbow without a little rain."
~ Unknown

As soon as my son talked, he asked for a baby sister. I wanted to give him that baby sister. I wanted a little girl, too. When he turned three, we told him he would be a big brother. He was so excited; we were happy. The climb up the roller coaster was always so exciting, but two months later, pulling him in the wagon back from our neighborhood pool, my stomach started cramping. I thought I was hungry. Once home, I took off my bathing suit and saw blood. With my first pregnancy, I had no issues and up to this point; I felt wonderful with this one, too. I wasn't too concerned. I thought I should do what the books say and call my doctor and elevate my legs.

"I'm sorry." If the doctor said anything else, I didn't hear it or remember it. I called one of my best friends and asked her, "What did he mean?" She was a sonographer who did lots of ultrasounds, even a few on this pregnancy. She told me to meet her at the hospital, we would see what was going on. We left our son with a neighbor and made our way to the hospital. My best friend had to tell me the baby's heart was no longer beating. My heart broke. That deep ache was so strong that I wasn't sure I could even make it out the door. But, I had to tell our little boy, Ryan, that I had miscarried. What I felt was that I had failed. I could not give him the baby sister he wanted. The next day I had a D & C. It was the hardest thing I had ever done. Gone were my chances of having a baby girl. I considered it my punishment for being bad—bad as a little girl and, now, a bad mom.

My doctor said more than once what I was going through was "normal." Miscarriages happen every day. It's just how it is. It wasn't my fault. I did nothing to cause it. The roller-coaster ride continued. I was put back on birth control[1] and dove into a depression; work was the only thing that got me up in the morning. My son became a chore and a reminder of my failure as a mom. I worked on myself. I started Body-for-Life[2] a 12-week nutrition and exercise program. Looking back, I can see how changing my diet and exercise helped bring me out of the depression, and then stopping the birth control helped me feel more like—me—the woman and mom I wanted to be. I was ready to try for a baby again. Maybe this time everything would be perfect.

We had our precious little girl—our *rainbow baby—a gift from God. I thought it righted everything. My life would be perfect. Now I had my boy and my girl—the perfect family of four. During each pregnancy and after each birth it was like I was on this roller coaster high—I wish I could put into words the difference in how I felt—the love, acceptance, excitement, adrenaline. It was a feeling I wanted to last forever.

*Rainbow Baby: a baby born after a miscarriage, stillbirth, or the death of an infant from natural causes.

GROWING FAMILY - DESERT STORM

"Make no mistake about it: Operation Desert Storm truly was a victory of good over evil, of freedom over tyranny, of peace over war."
~ Dan Quayle

It wasn't long after my daughter's birth that I felt like I was walking through the desert again. My kids weren't perfect, my marriage wasn't perfect. Our finances weren't perfect. I pretended everything was fine, but inside I was miserable. It was like another storm was raging within and I had no way to stop it. My husband and I went through marriage counseling. I thought our problems were his fault, but through counseling, I recognized it was me. I still couldn't share my past or how I felt about myself, but I saw my past was catching up with me, that hostility was leaking out, and hurting those I loved the most.

Then when my daughter was three, I got pregnant again. Something about me agrees with pregnancy. I feel fantastic pregnant. It's like my hormones are more balanced. I'm more balanced. I'm happy.

Our son and daughter were excited; they wanted to know if they would have a baby brother or a baby sister. We went to my best friend to do an ultrasound to see the sex of the baby. I already had an ultrasound at my doctor's office at 6 weeks and all was good. Now, at 12 weeks, she couldn't find the baby. It was like my seat dropped and I was falling or, more appropriate, I had failed again. What the world calls a miscarriage, the doctor calls "normal."

This time I would learn from this and not go into the depression I had gone into after my first miscarriage. I mean, I had a boy and a girl—the perfect life per the world's standards. This was just "normal." I pretended to be A-OK. That deep, dark hole in my heart had just gotten bigger—I would ignore and pretend it was not there. I would be the best wife, the best mom, the best friend.

I dealt with what I now know as anxiety, but at the time it just felt like this overwhelming heaviness all over—like an elephant was standing on my chest. It was this never-ending coaster spinning out of control.

Then I got pregnant again, and the fear of another miscarriage came with even more anxiety. I would do all I knew to make it go away. I would feed the anxiety with food. We had a beautiful little boy. Again, the first few months were wonderful. I was strong, confident, loving, and I could handle it all.

Have you dealt with anxiety and depression in your own life?
Have you tried to ignore the pain inside?
Have you looked to food to cover your pain?

"This was just "normal." I pretended to be A-OK."

3 KIDS- RUNAWAY TRAIN

"It is like trying to stop a runaway train
with one hand tied behind my back."
~ Katherine Alred

Now with three kids, homeschooling, working, and my hormones out of whack. Overwhelmed, exhausted, no energy was my normal.

I was 38 years old at the peak of my brokenness. I had a wonderful husband of seventeen years, three beautiful children—the oldest was the golden boy poster child and I expected nothing more than what I got from this wonderful young man. My daughter was beautiful, fun loving, and everything a mom could ever want in a little girl. My youngest son... one word has always fit him so well: cute!

So, what was wrong with me?
I had my yearly check-ups with my OB/GYN where I would share my hormonal and physical issues. I kept most of my emotional issues and feelings to myself. He was always great when I was pregnant and even made me feel good about myself when I had my miscarriages... "This is not your fault; it's all normal," but in everyday life, his answers just didn't match up.

How could this be "normal"?
Through the years he had given me every birth control pill (BCP) to help my acne, or stabilize my moods, or... to be honest, I'm not sure. I would complain that they made my skin crawl or made me feel crazy, or... one day after reading an article about the negative effects of birth control pills, including emotional/mental side effects, I decided they were not the best answer for me.[1] I told him my decision that I wanted no more BCP's.

He gave me some new recommendations—antidepressants or a hysterectomy. I didn't feel depressed. Looking back and learning more about all the different ways depression can feel, maybe I *was* dealing with depression. I lost two babies, and I had not allowed myself to grieve. I felt there was more. There had to be a reason, and I didn't feel either was the answer for me.

I saw so many other moms who went down that road, and from my view, their lives didn't seem any better for it. Some even seemed to be worse. Looking back, I remember moms talking at the park about the antidepressants prescribed to them, but I never remember another mom confiding in me about how she felt and why she was taking them. Maybe it was because I didn't confide in her. I was busy hiding behind my perfect "heads" life.

It was like we were all too afraid to share our past, about our fears, how we felt inside, but it was "normal" to tell the world about the little pill that the doctor said would change it all.

If you take antidepressant medication, please know that I do not think it is the wrong choice for you or that I'm judging you. I know that what you are feeling is real and the reason you are taking them is that you believe it is the best thing for you and your family. I hope you have people in your life you can talk to and share your feelings with.

I have spent the past ten years studying this topic and have found experts I trust. For me, antidepressants were not the answer and I'm happy I chose a different road.

My question then and still today is: *Why?*

- *Why* do we have these emotions and feel the way we feel?
- *Why* do we feel the pressures of the world are on us?
- *Why* are depression and anxiety considered normal?

Is there a root cause? Is there a more natural way to fix the problem rather than a drug or removal of body parts?

Regarding body parts... The other choice given to women in our culture is the hysterectomy. Did you know that *hysterical* meaning "affected by uncontrolled extreme emotion" comes from the Greek word for "in the womb?" Hysterectomies started in the Victorian Era to help women who had become hysterical. If the cause is the womb, let's remove it.

I am not the first to have felt the hormonal/emotional roller coaster syndrome, nor will I be the last. And I'm not sure how many women I have talked to through the years who were told to have a hysterectomy with the promise of it solving all of their problems. It never made sense to me. I had watched my mom and several ladies have hysterectomies at a young age, and it didn't appear to solve all their life problems—they just jumped on a new roller coaster.

As a physical therapist, I had listened to the additional problems these women were dealing with after the surgery caused by surgical menopause. So here it was 2009, and I was sick and tired of being sick and tired, and I felt like I was hiding it all pretty well. I appeared to be a good wife, homeschooling mom, successful physical therapist—you know, the typical American Superwoman. But, inside, all I could think of was; How can I run away from this perfect life that feels overwhelming and dark?

I decided my male doctor just did not understand—his solutions were from a man's perspective, and I needed a woman who could understand where I was coming from. I scheduled my appointment with the female "fixer-upper" doctor whom I had all the faith in the world would better understand me and would fix my physical issues, which would fix my emotional issues. Her assessment was the same as my male doctor—I was NORMAL. She did a few tests and sent me on my merry way.

Have you been given the "normal" diagnosis before?
How did it make you feel?

The seed of my journey was planted in my mind. I no longer wanted normal! *Normal is highly overrated.* I found out from those tests I was anemic, which led me to a pregnancy test, which led to, "I'm pregnant," and back to my male doctor.

BABY #6- AFTERSHOCK

"Like a great earthquake, once a great sorrow has hit your heart and razed
you to the ground, minor aftershocks move you no more."
~ Author unknown

I am awakened by an explosion, as if a bomb just went off, I jump up
and run, holding myself as if it's possible to stop the glass from shattering. My body has betrayed me again. I make it to the toilet and see
the remains. *How can this be?* Hysterical, screaming for help, my heart
aching as if broken into pieces. The adrenaline running through my
veins keeping me alive. As I look to my left, my husband is standing
there at the door in horror. I can only imagine what he thinks. My
thoughts tell me he wants to run. Who could blame him? How much
more can one man take? What about our three children on the other
side of the house, oblivious to the terror and blood stained carpets?
Knowing what I must do: pull it together, take every emotion, every
feeling, and bury it deep down. It takes just a moment. I am an expert
at hiding the hurt; I have been doing it for as long as I can remember.

He's waiting for my instruction. "Go get something to put it in." He
leaves. Alone, I wash myself off, change my clothes, wait. He hands me
the plastic yogurt container. I don't want to take it—I ask him to do it.
He says he can't. I *do* the hardest thing I have ever done—retrieve our
baby and lie him in the container and shut the lid. Wanting to hold
him, comfort him, examine every little finger and toe, knowing I can
not handle it, I can't look, I can't feel, I've got to be strong. We walk
to the car and I sit, numb with the container in my lap as my husband
takes us to the Emergency Room.

I had been lying on the bed bleeding for two hours; when I tried to
get up, I felt faint. My husband told the nurse I wasn't feeling well, and
we didn't feel that I could walk out. Her answer, "here's a wheelchair
and a prescription." He took me home, I was numb. I remember saying
to my neighbor who was watching our children, I had no physical pain.
Truthfully, I was left with this eerie feeling life had been sucked out of

me. All night long, all I could feel was the blood flowing out of me onto the blue pad below. I couldn't roll over or get up without feeling like I would faint. My thoughts going back to the beginning, reliving each step: I am a failure—failure as a wife, as a mom, as a human being. I am not worthy to live.

Morning came and my husband went to work to cancel his patients so he could take me to my doctor. My mom was worried; the kids were worried, and all I could do was lie in the bed and pray for them. I didn't want to cause their worry. I was supposed to be strong, healthy, and take care of them. Isn't that what a mom does?

When it came time to leave for the doctor, I refused. My husband tried to carry me, but my body went limp. There was no way he could carry me to the car. We phoned the doctor to tell him we'd have to wait and go the next day. The doctor said, "No—today!" My husband checked my blood pressure and could not get a reading. The doctor said, "call 911"—he did.

When the ambulance arrived to take me to the hospital, I was worried about what everyone would think. The EMT was worried about me. As he was trying to do everything, including putting electrodes on my chest "just in case," he reassured me. I asked if I should pray for myself. He said, "Yes!"

It was at that moment I realized I could die. I knew if I died, I would go to heaven. I knew if I died, the pain from living on earth would go away. I knew if I died, my family would be sad. I knew if I died, I would leave my kids without a mother. I decided at that moment to pray for myself. I decided my kids needed me, my husband needed me, my mom needed me. I needed to live, there was a reason God put me on this earth and I needed to live it out to the end.

I made it to the hospital but had lost so much blood they weren't sure how I was still awake or even alive. They had to start a blood transfusion before they could even take me into surgery to stop the bleeding.

I had been in the medical field for years. I heard of women bleeding to death and always thought, *How can people be so stupid?* I learned how easy it can be to not see what is right in front of you—I had gone into hemorrhagic shock and didn't even know it. My doctor saved my life. I will forever be grateful.

But again he told me it was "normal." As I lay on that hospital bed I wanted to scream—there was nothing "normal" about what I had just gone through. I laid in bed all night receiving blood, praying to God for answers to questions I didn't even know to ask.

Here I was 38, and I thought nothing could get worse. But let me tell you 39 was like the exponential of 38! No, I didn't have cancer; I wasn't dying. Nothing in my outside world changed. I still had the perfect life revolving around me, but inside I was hurting. I physically felt like crap. Headaches three out of four weeks a month, on edge, wanting to hide from life, yet too ashamed to let anyone know how I felt. Other people had real-world problems. A friend's daughter was dying of cancer; a neighbor girl my daughter's age was fighting cancer. Another neighbor lost her son at age three. He was the same age as my youngest son. My life was good. *How could I share how I was feeling when I was "normal"?* All of this had one positive effect in my favor. I was tired of the roller coaster ride. I WAS DONE WITH NORMAL.

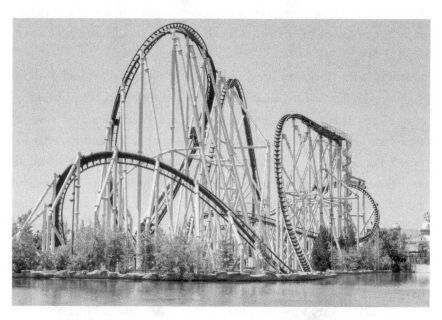

Do you feel you are on a roller coaster ride?

**Go to www.shawnacale.com/book-bonus
Printable Journal Pages and Bonus Resources
to Live an Exceptional Life.**

CHALLENGE: ROLLER COASTER RIDE

1. Take some time to journal about your own roller coaster ride.

2. Have you been told how you are feeling emotionally or physically is normal? How did it make you feel?

3. Have you ever been given a pill or something else as a quick solution and still feel there is something more: a better answer, a different solution?

4. What do you feel is at the core of your roller coaster ride?

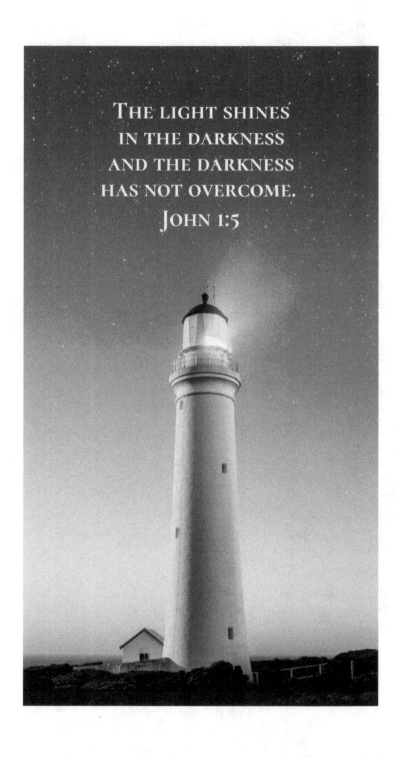

THE LIGHT SHINES
IN THE DARKNESS
AND THE DARKNESS
HAS NOT OVERCOME.
JOHN 1:5

3

The Healing Journey

Ask and it will be given to you; seek and you will find; knock and the door will be opened to you. For everyone who asks receives; the one who seeks finds; and to the one who knocks, the door will be opened.
~ Matthew 7:7-8 (NIV)

My search began. This one important lesson I had learned in my 39 years of life became my new focus. It's funny how when you set out for answers, opportunities appear to be everywhere. Even on rough days at work.

I was going over a new patient's chart and I noticed he was 10 years younger than me, and his list of medications added up to over twenty. How can one man not quite 30 years old be on so many medications? The truth is over 70% of American's are on medications.[1] Here's the thing: He was not the first patient I had seen with a long list of prescription medications—it was the norm. What surprised me most was he marked *good* as his health status.

Any other day I may have just ignored the whole scenario. But this day—my head was pounding, my body aching, and I was just going through the motions, counting the hours until I could go home and go to bed. If I had filled out a health form, I would have either marked *fair* or *poor*, and I had no medications or diagnosis to list.

His answers piqued my curiosity. I asked him more about his health. We talked about all his diagnoses and he told me how his high blood pressure, diabetes, and other long lists of issues were all managed with his prescriptions. His doctor had given him a *good* bill of health. How could that be? He was obese, just had shoulder surgery with a diagnosis of arthritis. How could he believe his health was *good*?

It made me want to cry—the question was: *Would the tears be for him or me?* Who was I to judge? I believed my overall health was *poor*. Time stopped for just a moment. What do I do with this information? Go back to my doctor and tell him to give me the antidepressants, the pain pills, have the surgery...

My thoughts flipped. Did he know the consequences of these drugs, his lifestyle choices? How could he believe his health was *good*? What lie was he living—whose truth was he believing? What would life be like in 10 years? His wife and four children sitting in the waiting room—would he be there for them? What kind of example was he setting for his family?

At that moment, I asked myself the same questions. It was like a light turned on and I understood in our society *good* was *normal*.

The word *exceptional* popped into my head. I'm not sure why. It wasn't a word common to my vocabulary. Maybe it had been my son's spelling word, or I had read it in a book, or maybe it was a whisper from God. All I know is the word *exceptional* now stuck in my head like a beacon, searching for it—not knowing what it was or what it meant. Just knowing there was more. I didn't have to follow the path that led to disease. I had hope.

> Exceptional now stuck in my head like a beacon.

THE VOLCANO

"If your heart is a volcano, how shall you expect flowers to bloom?"
~ Khalil Gibran

Just a few days later, I picked up *Natural Awakenings,* a magazine that was sitting on the table while having lunch at a new healthy restaurant. Inside was an ad: *Are you ready to get off the hormonal/emotional roller-coaster?* Yes! Just reading these words made me feel like someone out there understood me. Was this an answer from God?

She was a naturopath—a term I didn't know, so I googled it right there as I was eating my lunch. A *naturopath* focuses on long-term health and prevention. They can work with you to address a wide range of conditions, including gastrointestinal issues, stress and nervous tension, sleeplessness, fertility problems, headaches, joint health, and skin conditions. I thought, *Wow! She may have the answers I have been seeking.*

I checked her out and saw that she was a mom like me. She had dealt with some serious health issues and decided there was a better way. I told my wonderful husband what I had found. He had the typical financial questions: *Does she take insurance? How much will it cost?* "No" was the answer to insurance, and I told him the cost.

While he saw and lived with my outbursts, he did not understand how I felt inside because I didn't think I could confide in him. How do you tell your husband you love dearly that you spend hours thinking of ways to run away? I knew it wasn't him, and I didn't really believe it was the kids or my life. I didn't know what the problem was, which is why I thought maybe this naturopath could help me. He didn't think it was necessary, and the cost was too high. I was disappointed. I thought maybe she was the answer. I wasn't sure how much longer I could travel down this road. I knew something had to change.

Then one beautiful, yet not so pretty "Shawna" summer day, I was at the top of my hormonal/emotional rollercoaster and a volcano of words spewed out of my mouth and onto my husband. He received every bit of the burning lava.

I remember it like yesterday. He was outside by the trash cans. Who knows what I was mad about, but I went off on him and he just looked at me. It's like I can see the whole thing, like watching a movie. A scary movie. He had no words at first. Then it was like I woke up and realized what I was doing. I stopped. I wanted to be a wonderful wife, an excellent mom. I didn't want to scream and yell. I didn't want to feel the way I felt. I just stood there. He looked at me and said, "If that lady can help you, then go." Shame had now set in. I wondered if any of my neighbors heard me. Sure enough, people were outside. *What would they think?*

I knew I needed help. Before my husband could change his mind, I went inside and called to schedule an appointment.

THE NATUROPATH

"If you change nothing, nothing will change."
~ Joyce Brothers

It was Labor Day weekend; my appointment with the naturopath was just days away. I was excited to fill out all the paperwork. Kept a food diary for a week. I shared more than I had ever shared with another human being. When I reached my appointment, she began reviewing what I had written in my health history. She was understanding and believed together we could find the root cause. To be honest, by the end of my 3-hour consultation, I thought she was a little crazy. Maybe even crazier than my doctor who wanted to fix me with medications and surgical procedures.

She told me I just needed to change my lifestyle. *What?* I live the perfect life, with the perfect diet, with... I went home and read through the papers she had given me. I was living the "normal" American life. She called it SAD, and it stood for "Standard American Diet." She told me how the water I was drinking could be part of the problem. *What?* I prided myself on drinking plenty of water and teaching my patients how important water is to a healthy body. She gave me information on tap water and chlorine, bromine, fluoride. *What?* Fluoride could cause my problems—my toothpaste was bad, too. She told me low fat/no fat was harming my hormones and the cooking oil I used was detrimental to my health.

Every "healthy" food I had listed in my food diary, she told me what was wrong with it—I was eating way too much sugar. My idea of healthy eating was a bowl of cereal for breakfast that did not have sugar listed as the first ingredient because that is what my momma taught me. I had low-fat yogurt with real sugar and not aspartame for a snack because I knew artificial sweeteners gave me a headache. I had peanut butter and jelly on wheat bread and an orange for lunch because I knew white bread was bad. I had grilled chicken, salad with low-fat dressing, and potatoes for dinner. I mean, I was getting all the food groups by the end of the day. I treated myself to the occasional low-fat ice cream or pudding for dessert but, overall, I made excellent choices. No Twinkies, Ding-Dongs, or Pop-Tarts at *my* house!

My brain wanted to say, "Lady, you are wrong." But, my heart said, "If you want something different, Shawna, *do* something different." It was like the word *exceptional* was playing over and over in my mind. I listened to her. I wanted to be open to change, but could *my* choices be the reason for my problems?

My male doctor had always told me it wasn't my fault. It was all *normal.* The Naturopath was telling me I would need to take responsibility for my health and make these simple changes, and I would see amazing results. Two different philosophies. What was I to believe? Who was I to believe?

Have you ever gone looking for answers yet resisted change?

"If you want something different... do something different."

40 DAYS

"Food is thy medicine."
~ Hippocrates

My journey began. It was a slow process. I started with a water filtration system. I noticed fewer headaches but figured it was more of a coincidence than a result. That was until we went on vacation and I drank regular tap water. I got a headache that day. *Could it make that big of a difference?* We bought filtered water and no headache the next day. I used coconut oil to cook with and on my body instead of lotion. *Could my acne be going away?*

I decided 40 days before my 40th birthday I would do the *Maker's Diet*[2] by Jordan Ruben, a book the naturopath had recommended. I would go ALL in and see if what she said was true. I didn't believe my diet was the culprit, but I was happy to prove her wrong and move on to the next recommendation. Instead, my life was shaken upside down. This diet was a low to no-sugar diet, which I thought would not be a problem since we didn't keep a lot of sweets in the house. Boy, was I wrong!

By day five, I was miserable, cranky, shaky, and ready to quit. I felt worse than ever. By noon I was in my room hiding out from my kids—protecting them from any hurtful words that may spew from my mouth. When my husband came home, I looked like a person you would see on a rehab reality show. I was curled up in a ball and shaking. All I could think was how ridiculous it was for me to feel this way. *I should feel better. This shouldn't be that hard. What's wrong with me?*

Have you ever tried to do the right thing and thought you got the wrong result?

"I didn't believe my diet was the culprit, but I was happy to prove her wrong..."

He asked me what was wrong.

"I feel worse; this isn't working."

He said come watch a movie or play a game with the family.

"You don't want to be around me right now."

He said, "Go for a walk."

"I don't want to go for a walk."

He would not let me lie there, so I got up angrily, and I put on my shoes and walked out the door.

Now, I live on the best street in our neighborhood—lots of wonderful families and kids. As parents we raised our children together, we lived life together; we were there for each other in good times and in hard times. I also kept my inner me hidden from even my best friends and neighbors, and with time found out I was not the only one hiding secrets. I believed if people knew me, they would never like me. The lies we tell ourselves are real.

Since it was a beautiful Friday night, everyone was outside playing and enjoying the evening. I was in no mood to sit and talk, so I hurried past everyone to get off my street as fast as I could. On my way back, one of the young girls asked if I would like a cupcake. *Do you know the little mini bite-size cupcakes that you can pop into your mouth with one bite?* That's what she was offering me. I looked down the street and my family was nowhere in sight. They were the only ones who knew I was doing this diet. So, I said, "Yes!" I took it all in one bite and it felt heavenly. It was as if the rush of sugar coursed through my body and gave me a moment of happiness. It was only a moment because in just a short time I realized the dread was back. I walked to my house with a new awakening. I was a sugar addict.

How could I be a sugar addict? When did this happen? Could the naturopath be right? Could my choices be part of the problem? I wondered if sugar was the root cause of so many of my issues. Was there really that much-hidden sugar in my everyday life? Did I go to sugar to comfort my nerves? I was no longer in denial. I walked straight to my computer, and I typed up this poem...

I Am an Addict

Today, I realized I am an addict
I felt I should stand up and say
My name is... and I am an addict

But in today's world
We hide our addictions
Our shame keeps us quiet

I am not sure when I became an addict
I can't remember a time that I didn't enjoy
The feeling I received from my addiction

It started with just special occasions
Or maybe a little on the weekends

Then it became a treat that was deserved daily
For all the hard work I had done
Then it was more of a habit
Something to do when bored or lonely

My habit became more difficult to control
It became a daily desire, a need

It couldn't be an addiction
Because if I wanted to stop, I could stop
I just wasn't ready

Then I was ready to make a change
Become a new me
Today, I would break the habit

A week went by with nothing
The thrill of breaking the habit
Should have been enough

Instead, headaches, shaking, tears
Feelings of going crazy, skin-crawling
And wanting to run far away

I thought to break the habit
Would make life easier
But no, it made life unbearable

Trying to stay away from temptation
When it was lurking around each and every corner
Kept me on my toes

Then the moment happened.
"Would you like some?"
Instead of saying "No"
I took from the forbidden fruit.

I wish I could say,
It was awful, but it wasn't
The feeling that occurred in one second
The high from the hit,
Was fantastic

In moments the feeling was gone,
The guilt replaced it quickly
But, that is when I realized
I am an addict

by Shawna Cale

ADDICTIONS

"When you can stop you don't want to,
and when you want to stop, you can't..."
~ Luke Davies

Oh, that's not so bad. Everyone eats sugar. Sugar doesn't ruin lives as alcohol does. It doesn't kill like cigarettes. Sugar doesn't hurt others like illegal drugs. The lie I believed for almost 40 years. Looking back, I see how sugar can destroy and how it could have destroyed me.

I still desire sugar, but I no longer use the words, "I love sugar" or, "I can't live without sugar." I do my best to *not* buy white sugar and bring it into my house; that's my safe place. Occasionally I will have it out in public or at a family gathering. I use more natural sweeteners to help curb my sugar cravings, and I find I don't crave it like I used to. Instead, I crave nuts. I can't pass by a nut without eating it. If given a choice between a cupcake and a cup of nuts, I would ask if I could have both, because the two together would be heavenly. If allowed only one, I hope I would pick the nuts, but that is a journey I am still walking.

Are there things in your life you feel you cannot give up or stop?

Or, perhaps like me, you have been living in denial. Maybe it's time to ask yourself: *Is there something I choose that is not good for my health?* It's very freeing to admit. Like any addiction, it is not an easy road, but I welcome you to start on the journey with the rest of us. You won't regret it.

The day after I realized my addiction, I spent the next 35 days learning whatever I needed to learn about myself through this experience. I wish I could say that it was easy, but with each step, it was less difficult. I was understanding why I turned to food. Sweets made me feel better—at that moment. I studied, went to classes, listened to videos, and learned about health in a new way. I learned about functional medicine, holistic health, and what wellness was—and it wasn't the checkup I took my kids to yearly.

Within the first 30 days, I saw results. One morning as I was walking into my bedroom, I felt this warmth in my panties. I thought one of two things just happened—I just peed my pants or I just started my period. Mortified to think I could have peed in my pants just walking through the house, but I had no signs of starting my period. I never needed to keep a calendar or anything to let me know when my next cycle started because I had a headache three days before my period ever since I was thirteen years old. I went to the bathroom and realized I had my first ever "exceptional" period. I say that because this period was not "normal" this period felt different, it looked different. No headache at all that week. The blood was a bright red and a thin consistency instead of a dark, clotty black color. I did not have cramps, backache, or feel pissed off every minute of the day. I had not been dreaming about how I could run away. The changes in my diet changed my period, not just that month, but every month since.

I completed those 40 days and decided I was ready to be the unusual one, making food from scratch, sprouting grain, eating fresh fruits and vegetables, making homemade bread—not the typical way for the "normal" American family. What I found is that I was changing—what I was doing from the outside was making a change on the inside. My once "normal" life was feeling exceptional.

Have you ever thought what you eat could affect how you feel?

"Within the first 30 days, I saw results."

WHITE FLOUR TORTILLA EFFECT

"Do you think it was the white flour tortilla?"
~ Kevin Cale

I had completed my 40-day journey the day before my 40th birthday. I was now 5 pounds lighter and felt like I had released 50 pounds of emotional baggage. I was ready to feel this way forever and live this new life committed to the changes I had made.

My family celebrates holidays and celebrations around food and they wanted to take me out to eat at our favorite Mexican restaurant. I ordered a salad, had a few tortilla chips and salsa. I *knew* I would say "no" to the sopapilla. I felt good, I was happy to be with my family, I was enjoying my birthday. As everyone was eating their sweet treat, I thought ONE white flour tortilla would be fine. I mean, it's my birthday, and how much sugar can be in one tortilla?

The next morning was a Sunday, and I was cleaning the house. I went back to my daughter's room and opened the door to a mess. I yelled at her; she cried. I could feel the anger building up within—I was mad! She knew it. My husband rushed to see what all the commotion was—the hero to save the day. I then told him all about it. How she *made* me so mad. Her room was a mess, and she hadn't done her chores. She is crying, and in her defense, yelling back, "My room is always a mess. That's the way I like it!" I'm shaking my head, thinking my husband is on my side until he utters these words: "Do you think it was the white flour tortilla?" Never ask a woman if it's that time of the month when she is having a PMS moment and do not ask a woman if what she ate the night before was causing her to behave irrationally. She will only get more ticked off.

I stomped off to my room with those words repeating in my mind like a broken record: *Could it have been the white flour tortilla?* One white flour tortilla could not have been the cause. It wasn't me; it was her. If she just did what I asked and cleaned her room, everything would be good, I would not have yelled at her.

What if it *was* the white flour tortilla? What if it *was* what I ate that caused me to spiral out of control? I laid there in my bed crying. I wanted to be a wonderful mom, an excellent wife. I thought I was better. I thought changing my diet for 40 days "fixed" me. I felt so good the day before, now I felt awful—physically *and* emotionally. After crying, I got up, walked to my daughter's room, and apologized. I told her I didn't want to yell and scream, but I wanted her to keep her room clean. She told me I hadn't yelled at her for over a month and her room was a mess then... Why today?

I contemplated that question for a long time. After going for spurts with no sugar, white flour, fast food I would find I could handle so much more of life, but one white flour tortilla, a piece of birthday cake, a brownie, a muffin, a donut... the littlest bit would set me off. It would throw me right back onto the hormonal/emotional roller coaster that had been my "normal" for so long.

I would have never believed the difference food could make to my hormones and emotions without feeling the effects myself. Often, we think we can handle just one bite, one drink, one pill. For me, it was "just" sugar. It wasn't a crime. I wasn't doing anything everyone else wasn't doing. I looked around, I saw the damage. The damage it was causing to my health. The damage it was causing in my relationships.

I will always have a propensity toward sugar. Most days I say "no" without a problem. The longer I abstain, the easier it becomes, but sometimes I say "yes," and the consequences always follow. I feel like crap. My joints hurt, my head aches, and my outbursts hurt those I love most.

I am learning and growing and understanding myself more every year. I believe milestone moments help us grow and peel back the layers to see who God created us to be. I look at my failures now with new-found hope. I had felt the difference. I continued to ask questions. I continued to wait and listen for answers. I was no longer looking for a destination. I was on a healing journey.

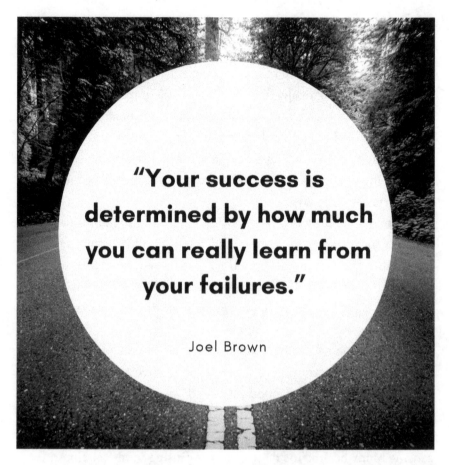

"Your success is determined by how much you can really learn from your failures."

Joel Brown

Go to www.shawnacale.com/book-bonus
Printable Journal Pages and Bonus Resources
to Live an Exceptional Life.

CHALLENGE: ADDICTIONS

1. List any "addictions" that could prevent you from having the health you desire?

2. Spend some time thinking and journaling about the addictions you listed and how they may affect your spiritual, emotional, and physical health and those you love.

4

Milestone Moments

"The only time we can fail is if we quit.
Most perceived failures are only stepping-stones
being small problems encountered along the path to a goal.
Obstacles are opportunities for growth, therefore,
encourage and embrace them."
~ Arthur Frederick Saunders

As I grew, I realized that the outside work—changing my diet and getting rid of toxic products was not the hard work. It was the inside that still needed to change, to move toward living an exceptional life. I wish I had a quick recipe for success because I know that is what so many people seek—the average, normal way of living life. The exceptional life is living day by day, learning and growing while on your journey.

In this season I was feeling like I had awakened from a 40-year journey in the desert and my gift was the Promised Land. Every day was a fresh start, a stone appearing leading me in the direction I was to go.

One morning, in January 2011, I woke up with what I can best explain as a vision from God: the answer to the questions I had been asking, "How do I improve my health? How do I live an exceptional life?"

I may have dreamed of what I will share with you while I was sleeping, but most of the experience happened when I was awake—it was my letter on the wall.

I grabbed a pen and a thin piece of cardboard that had been sitting on my nightstand and wrote: Ex S E P s h N L Health. *Each day we will begin to look at the different areas of our life and begin to make some changes. Remember, there must be action or no change will occur.*

I knew God had given me these letters as an acronym or mnemonic. It was as if I was a detective as I wrote each letter down, one by one, and asking the Lord what each one meant. Then I read it from left to right—it was exceptional!

Can I be real with you? I was excited—for about 10 minutes. Excited because God had answered my questions and even gave me a formula. But then I felt the "calling."

Have you ever felt *called*?

I knew what it was because I felt it when He *called* me to be a physical therapist as a junior in high school. Then He *called* me to homeschool when my oldest son was in the second grade. Now, He was asking me to share with the world what He had just given me. He planted this seed to write a book, and I wasn't even sure what it was about.

I questioned, "Lord, who would I give this to? Who would listen to me?" Yes! That was fear and not faith speaking. Looking back, I still had a lot of growth, but now I know that growth would have happened if I had listened and followed His lead. Instead, I argued and looked for my own answers.

Would you believe I said, "Lord, people won't believe this is from you if Ex= *exercise* and comes before *spiritual.*" I continued, "Lord, don't you know lots of Christians don't like the word *spiritual.*" "Who would read my book?" Yes, I was arguing with God.

Have you ever argued with God?

I know I am not the only one. In the Bible, there are several accounts of men and women arguing with God. Moses told God he couldn't tell Pharaoh to let his people go because he wasn't a good speaker—he was slow of speech and tongue.[1] Sarah laughed when she heard she was to have a baby at an old age.[2] Me, I wasn't a writer. We often find excuses when things look hard.

Now, I wrote everything I heard Him say, and I spent time every day researching every aspect, and I even looked at what He gave me and made a checklist, thinking this must be what I am supposed to do. I thought if I do everything daily, I will have better health and be living an exceptional life. Then I can tell the world...

IBUPROFEN

"Success is a process. During that journey sometimes there are stones thrown at you, and you convert them into milestones."
~ Sachin Tendulkar

I love how God orchestrates just what we need at the right time. I had patients at the physical therapy clinic asking me questions about their pain medications and what was better over-the-counter... ibuprofen or Tylenol, or the pain medications the doctor prescribed. Pharmacology was my least favorite class in school. I didn't like to take medications because most of the time they made me feel worse instead of better, but I had my favorite: ibuprofen. It was my friend. I kept it with me at all times, and most days I took it 2-3 times. Either I needed it for a headache, leg ache, backache, or cramps. It was my go-to for all things until...

I had a patient ask me if I knew anything about ibuprofen causing problems with cartilage.[3] *What?* "No! I have never heard of such a thing!" I am a research nerd at heart. I did some digging and found a few articles on the damage ibuprofen could cause. This was a tough moment for me because a doctor had once told me that keeping inflammation down by using something like ibuprofen could prevent my arthritic symptoms from getting worse. I had a goal of never having to have a knee, hip, or any other joint replaced. I had watched far too many surgeries and treated hundreds of patients. I was all about prevention and now I read that my go-to could cause damage. I remember when ibuprofen became an over-the-counter drug, and it was a good day in my book. Now, I would have to decide between saying "yes" to pain or "yes" to something that may cause damage. *How do you make that kind of decision?*

I did more research. I researched food for joint pain. My headaches and cramps were almost obsolete at this point in my journey with the changes I had made, but I continued to have joint pain. I found bone broth may be a good option and began making it. I wanted to know all I could learn about nutrition and how it could help me and my patients instead of pharmaceuticals.

As a homeschooling mom, I went every year to the Oklahoma Homeschool Convention with one of my best friends, and I was excited to go learn about a curriculum called *Nutrition 101*... how great it would be to teach my children what I had been learning. It is now May 2011; I am sitting in the *Nutrition 101* class when the woman teaching talks about essential oils. I do not understand what oils she is talking about. In the past 9 months, I had learned about coconut oil, olive oil, and all the problems with products such as Crisco and Wesson cooking oil. I asked what aisle I would find essential oil at the grocery store since she had so many exceptional things to say about it. She kind of laughed and told me she would tell me more at her table.

When I walked up to the table, I did not know what I was getting myself into. I told her about my current health journey, and she shared an earful of information on all the outstanding things about essential oils and her story, too. I thought this was too good to be true, but I had seen what changing my diet had done for my health, so I listened. She then brought up how essential oils are in the Bible. *What?* I had read through my Bible from front to back at least five times and couldn't remember essential oils being mentioned. This concept intrigued me. I told her that most restaurant foods gave me a headache and that my head was hurting from the lunch I had earlier. I was doing my best to make choices that limited my need for ibuprofen and was no longer keeping it in my pocket or close by. She told me she had a solution. She gave me a drop of a special blend, a drop of Frankincense (*what they gave Jesus?*), and a drop of Peppermint, showing me how to inhale each one and put it on my neck and temples. She continued to talk, and my head continued to ache. I'm sure half of what she said went in one ear and out the other. I walked away from the table without a lot of faith in drops of oils, taking my headache away.

I wondered what people might think as they smelled me when they passed by me. My friend asked me how my head was feeling? I said, "It hurts. I will need to go back to the hotel before the next session to get some ibuprofen." We walked farther, and she asked, "Are you ready to go back to the hotel?" I looked at her surprised and said, "It's gone, but it will be back." I figured it took about 20 minutes to work and that's how long it took for the effects of ibuprofen to kick in—could this be a solution? In the past with ibuprofen, my headaches always returned a few hours later, requiring more ibuprofen.

Back in the hotel room that evening, we stayed up talking until 2 a.m. and my headache never came back. "Lord, is this another answer to another prayer?"

The next morning, I went back to that same table and found out the price of the essential oils. I was prepared to buy books for the next school year, not to spend $150 on voodoo oils, even if they had worked this one time. I saw a book called *Healing Oils of the Bible*[4] by Dr. David Stewart and decided that would be a great place to start. I love books. I love to read. I read the book from cover to cover in less than 48 hours. I had never realized all the things in the Bible that were related to our health.

> "Lord, is this another answer to another prayer?"

"You love righteousness and hate wickedness; therefore God, your God, has set you above your companions by anointing you with the oil of joy."
PSALM 45:7 (NIV)

I started researching essential oils and stopped taking ibuprofen. Again, it was amazing how many things came my way to help with my pain once I gave up my drug of choice. I paid attention to my food and how I felt the day after. I took Epsom salt baths and after three months of research and buying my first essential oils kit[5]; I found food, oils, and supplements could meet all the needs I used ibuprofen for in the past, except now it was not that big of an issue since the pain was occasional and not daily. I had not felt so good in I don't know how many years, if *ever*.

In 2012, I began blogging about ExSEPshNL™ health and wellness, and put together a little email course, and had a few people go through it. But something was missing. The letter "E" for *emotional* had me stumped. I knew emotional health was important, but I believed the only change that could occur for a person was from a physical aspect. When circumstances in the world were excellent—emotions excellent. Feeding my body nutritious food—emotions excellent. Exercise, enough good water, and sleep and emotions were excellent. Everything came from the physical side.

THE INTENSIVE

"I've discovered that every time I've reached a milestone I think I'm there, but there's another there waiting for me."
~ Sara Benincasa

It was March 2012, so many pieces of the ExSEPshNL puzzle seemed to be missing, I was searching for answers. Asking more questions. *How could I write a book on a formula that I still didn't completely understand?*

It was then that I was invited to a class called the *Raindrop*[6]. I did not know what it was, but I was eager to learn. I entered the building and a woman I had met the week before told me I would go to a CARE Intensive[7]. I wasn't sure what she was talking about—a *CARE Intensive*? She was telling me all about it and how it was taking place during Spring Break out of town. *Stop*. I knew I would not be going to this event. I was working for my husband at the Physical Therapy Clinic so he could take our oldest son to the National Homeschool Basketball Championships. She continued to tell me I was going, yet I knew it was impossible.

Names went into a drawing for this free Raindrop technique and they drew my name. I still did not understand what a Raindrop was, except that it was a bunch of oils they would put on my feet and then on my back. As I lay on the massage table, a man named Max gave me the Raindrop as his wife Karen—the woman who introduced me to oils at the homeschool convention—explained to the audience what he was doing. I felt amazing; you know the moment between being awake and asleep, that's where I was at. Everyone wanted to know what I thought about it. As I sat on the edge of the table, I felt like a backpack with a ton of bricks had been lifted off my back and I didn't even know I'd been carrying it. I found out that the CARE Intensive was a three-day class where people learn about the Healing Oils of the Bible, the Chemistry of essential oils, VitaFlex, Raindrop, and Emotional Release.

At home, I told my husband all about the experience... the woman telling me I would go to this CARE Intensive, receiving the Raindrop, feeling amazing as if I was light as a feather and walking on clouds, and all about what CARE entailed... my house phone rang. It was Max on the other end: "We have a scholarship we would like to offer you for the CARE Intensive coming up... Would you be interested?" I'm sure I was standing there with my mouth wide open. I had to work Friday, but I could do Saturday and Sunday. He told me it had to be the full three days. *What could I do?* I told him I would let him know. Praying as I walked back to my husband and shared with him the conversation. He made what seemed like an impossible phone call to find someone to cover for me at work on Friday. She said, Yes! It felt like a miracle. I called Max back with my reply: a resounding "Yes!"

That weekend would change the course of my life in so many ways. I could see God's hand in every step I took, but what happened on the last day changed me in a way that I could have never expected. I felt from the moment I walked into the hotel I was there for a reason. The facilitators walked us through what the three days would look like and said that somebody on the last day would receive an Emotional Release. I didn't know what that meant, but I knew I didn't want it to be me.

They call it an "intensive" for a reason. It was an intense three days of learning and putting what you learn into action. The right side of my back was hurting off and on all weekend, but by the third morning, I was in pain. After lunch, it was time to learn more about releasing emotions that no longer serve us. *What does that even mean?* I didn't know how my emotions served me or didn't serve me. It confused me and was out of my comfort zone. I understood the physical body. I loved the Chemistry of Oils class... it made sense, but releasing emotions? That sounded a bit too woo woo to me.

They divided us into groups and told us to look through a book called *Releasing Emotional Patterns with Essential Oils*[8] by Carolyn Mein, D.C. to find an emotion that we were feeling or dealing with at the moment. When I have been introduced to something new or something I do not understand I become sarcastic. It's a protection mechanism. It's not the side of me I wanted people to see. But I did not understand how to put a word to how I was feeling, right there on the spot. I mean, maybe I felt that this was a stupid exercise? But, "stupid" did not appear to be an emotion in the book. I went through the list of emotions with not the best attitude, and I just didn't understand the concept. Then someone said that if I couldn't find an emotion and if there was an essential oil that I didn't like, it could mean that the emotion connected to it was something I might need to release. More confusion set in. Sure, there were several oils I didn't like the smell of—one of them being lavender. I looked at the emotions connected to lavender and though each of those was areas I had hidden issues with—I had no connection with my emotions to even have the awareness that I needed to let them go.

They then instructed us to look at pictures in the back of the book. If we had pain anywhere it could be emotional, and we could see if we could find the pain (alarm point) in the pictures. The picture showed the exact location of my back pain—marked "PSIS." I had been dealing with back pain at my Posterior Superior Iliac Spine (PSIS) since I was 21 years old, my first year of marriage, while in physical therapy school. I had spent almost two decades having other therapists, including my husband, try to fix my problem with no luck. Every continuing education course I ever took was to help my back—no change. Nobody could ever find anything wrong with it, but it hurt often. I found Pilates helped me manage the pain, but it never "fixed" the problem. I considered it my "thorn" in my side because I helped hundreds of people with back pain using the techniques I had learned, even though none of them worked for me.

Here I am, looking at this book and this so-called alarm point, and was told to find the emotion and oil connected to the location. The oil was myrrh. Yes, the same myrrh from the Bible given to Baby Jesus. The emotion: *difficulty*. At first, I thought, I don't think there is anything difficult here—my sarcasm, my I-am-always-right attitude, my ego... were all shining. Then I took a step back and thought, these three days have been difficult; it had shaken up most of what I believed about the medical field, along with the healing wonders I had seen in the room as participants used the techniques on each other.

I took the myrrh and was told to place it on the alarm point, inhale it and then exhale as I release "difficulty," and embrace the other side, which in this case was "knowing." The *way out* or what I like to call the affirmation was "I move with life." Now I thought, This is ridiculous. I will rub this oil on my back, smell it and say these words I don't even understand, and it's supposed to heal my back when 20 years of physical therapy and exercises have done very little. Talk about resistance; it was as thick as glue. I said the words, "I move with life." Rolled my eyes, "How many times am I supposed to say this?" "Until you believe it." "Then we might be here all night." I say, "I move with life" a second time and then a third. That's when something happened. I can't even explain it. I asked, "How long does it take for the pain to go away?" The answer I received was everyone is different. I wasn't sure I wanted to admit out loud my pain had disappeared, but no right lower back pain—it was as if it had never existed. I had to ask, "What just happened?" "You just released an emotion trapped, stored, being held in that part of your body." *Had I been given this opportunity to attend CARE for this moment? Did God want me to experience the healing that I never even knew was possible? Could an emotion have been causing me this issue all these years?* So many questions, yet so much gratitude.

It was then time to put our names into the drawing for an Emotional Release, where someone would lie on a table and walk through a process similar yet different from what we had just experienced on our own. I was reluctant to fill out the paper. Yet, I knew there was more for me to experience here. My name went into the bucket. We all sat down and a fear that they would choose me rose within. This wonderful woman, Carrie, whom I had just met that weekend, looked me in the eye and smiled as she held a piece of paper in her hand. *Was she looking at me, or was it the person behind me?* I wanted to turn around to look. But she just nodded her head when I looked at her as if she were saying, *it's you.* I cried. I don't cry, okay... I don't cry often. An enjoyable book, a wonderful movie, or a life crisis, but day-to-day I am not a crier, in public I DO NOT CRY. She announces my name, and I am told it's okay. This will be a beautiful experience. My stomach is in knots, I stand up.

My biggest fear was that something would come out I didn't want the world to know. You know... the stories I told you I had told no one before. I am lying on the massage table as Max is grounding my feet and Karen explains to the students what they were doing. Carrie, to my right, is whispering about the process she will walk me through. She hands me an oil and has me repeat after her. It took only a few minutes for me to feel safe and comfortable. A few more minutes and I was so relaxed that I didn't even know who else was in the room. Carrie walked me through, releasing the stored emotions I had with each baby I had lost. She asked me their names, and it was in these sweet moments I released grief, sadness, hate, and other emotions I had buried deep, deep inside.

I remember wailing as I had never wailed before. It was such a deep groan from so far within I didn't even recognize the sound. This time the wailing wasn't a holding it all in, but a release of what I had endured, and not released in my life. It was like I was free to just let it all go. I had never felt so much freedom in crying and I understood the concept of letting go of that which no longer served me as I went through the experience.

At one point I heard the words, "Shut up Karen" and I realized there was talking going on in the room, but I felt at peace as Carrie continued to walk me through the process. When it was over, I sat up on the edge of the table. In the past when I cried, I would have a terrible headache and feel like I needed to throw up, but this was different.

The group asked me questions, and I answered the best I could, "I felt light, carefree." I turned to look at Max and giggled, "I remember Max telling Karen to shut up." As everyone in the room looked from Max to Karen and laughed along with me. Max said that he never said it, but everyone knew he had been thinking it.

That day my life changed for a second time. The first was when I accepted Christ as my Lord and Savior at age 10. Now, 30 years later, I understand the power of emotions—the strongholds they can have on us and how they affect our lives. I may spend the rest of my life releasing emotions, but knowing I can release emotions that no longer serve me is a gift I will always cherish.

"Could an emotion have been causing me this issue all these years?"

BYE BYE NORMAL

"Normality is a paved road: It's comfortable to walk,
but no flowers grow on it."
~ Vincent van Gogh

Every morning when I awake, I have choices. Some say we make 35,000 choices a day. We make a choice about every 2.5 seconds we are awake. It's easy to take the normal road. It takes courage, time, and energy to choose the exceptional road.

In 2013, my mantra was, "Obedience is mine. Outcome is God's." I repeated this often when making a choice. I made some monumental steps that led me down a road that has changed my future. I began working on releasing emotions daily, more time in prayer, more walks, and more gratitude. I started a home-based business that brought me home full-time with my children in 2014. A dream I had but was too scared to live—faith was now taking over the fear. Being home gave me time with my family, time with friends, and I slowly started feeling it was safe to be me. I even had opportunities to travel the world, and in 2019 we bought our dream RV and traveled the USA.

I wish I could say I always choose the exceptional road, but I am human—not perfect. I wake up and the normal road is there waiting for me. Some days I find myself on it more than others. Often, my limiting beliefs get in my way and negative thoughts ruminate in my head. Trapped emotions or my feelings of the day often hold me captive. Other times I am traveling down the exceptional road, finding beauty and splendor all around me—taking thoughts captive and giving them to God. And then there are the times I find a roadblock—and I am stuck feeling no movement at all.

Roadblocks appear to be these huge circumstances we have no control over and stand in our way. What I have learned is that finding solutions for every roadblock is why God gave me the ExSEPshNL Formula for living out dreams, reaching goals, and my God-given purpose.

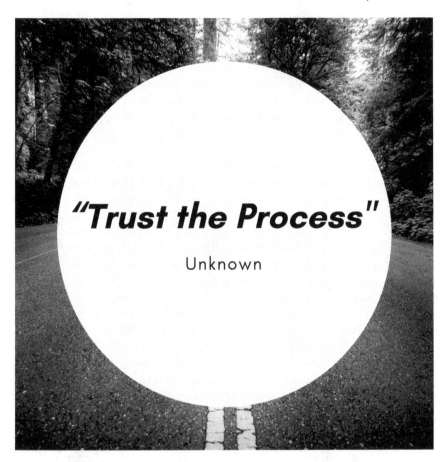

My husband and oldest son often say, "Trust the process." When trust is an issue that's often difficult to do, but that's what the Lord has taught me as He has walked with me, guiding me and showing me the exceptional way.

God even put people in my path—friends, coaches, programs that taught me steps to take to move past the roadblocks and reach the goals set before me. I thought for so long I needed to walk the exceptional road alone. As if it would take away from my quest by needing help and guidance. In 2017, I needed help and decided that working with a coach was the next step. I have had one or more coaches in my life for areas I need to grow ever since. One day after talking to my coach Gwen in 2018, I realized I was still trying to live my life from the outside in, basing my happiness, my self-worth, on my accomplishments. I told her about my *calling* to write a book. She told me my story needed to be told. I needed to share my gift with the world. I started. I stopped. Fear had set in.

I love how God can move right through a roadblock. In November 2018, my good friend Sunshyne and I were doing some personal development and planning for 2019. I went to bed and had a dream about my book being published on January 20, 2020. It would be the 10th anniversary of my traumatic experience and the day I decided my life was worth living.

I knew then my childhood trauma—the pain I had suffered, and the triumph found would forever live in a book—to bring value to the world. However, I was still seeking—joy in my daily life. So God planted a new coach in my life. One that led me down a road of additional questions, answers, more coaches, and love.

On July 20th, 2019, I let go of expectations, fears, and negative thoughts and I announced to the world or at least my little world—"I am writing a book."

I have realized living an exceptional life is about living from the inside out. That acronym I received from God almost ten years ago continues to be like a treasure map—checkpoints to lead me towards being who I am in this journey called "life." I am now thankful that by sharing my story I am not a victim of my childhood, but a victor who has shared her past and shown the world there is nothing that can prevent us from living the exceptional life—but ourselves.

I have one request before we move forward together, and I know it's a big one: Don't expect perfection from yourself or anyone else. In this book, I have shared my stories and in Part II I will give you the ExSEPshNL Formula in its entirety. Don't quit. The day-to-day failures do not make you a failure. It's the moment you get back up and say, "Bye bye normal, hello exceptional" that leads you to your goal—holistic health—an exceptional life.

Go to www.shawnacale.com/book-bonus Printable Journal Pages and Bonus Resources to Live an Exceptional Life.

CHALLENGE: CHOICES

1. What choices have you been making towards your goals?

2. What choices have you been making that lead you down the road you don't want to go?

3. What choice, no matter how small, can you take right now to living an exceptional life?

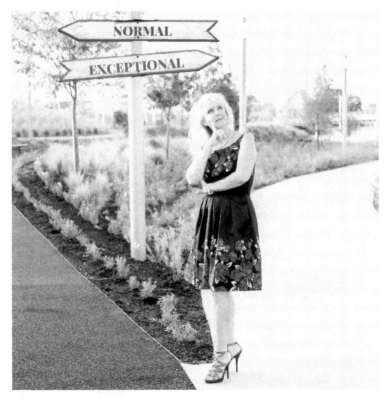

Living an Exceptional Life- One Choice at a Time
Sonja Marie Photography

PART 2

The Roadmap

Hello Exceptional

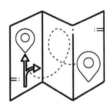

"Without a map, every road looks promising...
With a map, the right road becomes obvious."
~ Unknown

5

The ExSEPshNL Formula

"The question is not whether the formula for success will work,
but rather whether the person will work the formula."
~ Jim Rohn

Each of us has a story. I shared with you mine. There is much you can learn from your story, too. Your story got you where you are today; it is the road that you have traveled. However, your story is not who YOU are—it does not define you. Yes, your story played a part in creating the beliefs directing your results. But how often do we look back and realize our direction was not clear? We didn't know what roads to follow or actions to take.

Understanding my story helped me figure out what was blocking my path to holistic health, and it wasn't a lack of time, my eating habits, stress, or lack of exercise. It was deeper.

If you struggle with emotional or physical pain, are overweight, stressed out, worn out, anxious, depressed, fatigued the ExSEPshNL Formula provides solutions so you can walk the path that releases emotional triggers and traumas, excess weight, eases pain, and gives you the energy to do the things you love to do.

I want you to understand you are much more than your story. Are you ready for the best part? Your story is still being written. You are the CEO of your life and you get to decide every day the road you want to take to lead your story in the direction you choose.

The morning I awoke and wrote the letters ExSEPshNL was the day that I understood my choices are writing the story of my life. The beacon to live the exceptional life gave me a direction much like a lighthouse both warns and directs ships on the ocean. I would like to share with you the road map full of treasures I believe God gave me to direct my journey and to share with others to give hope and a future that points to a relationship with God and holistic health.

My desire then and today is to live an exceptional life.

The Tree of Life

What delight comes to the one who follows God's ways!
He won't walk in step with the wicked, nor share the sinner's way, nor
be found sitting in the scorner's seat.
His pleasure and passion is remaining true to the Word of "I Am,"
meditating day and night in the true revelation of light.

He will be standing firm like a flourishing tree planted by God's
design, deeply rooted by the brooks of bliss,
bearing fruit in every season of his life.
He is never dry, never fainting, ever blessed, ever prosperous.
But how different are the wicked.
All they are is dust in the wind-driven away to destruction!

The wicked will not endure the day of judgment, for God will not
defend them. Nothing they do will succeed or endure for long, for they
have no part with those who walk in truth.
But how different it is for the righteous!
The Lord embraces their paths as they move forward
while the way of the wicked leads only to doom.

- PSALM CHAPTER 1 (TPT)

EXCEPTIONAL HEALTH

"You can't be great if you don't feel great.
Make exceptional health your #1 priority.
~ Robin Sharma

I love to go on what I call a "walk and talk." It's funny how when you walk and talk you let your guard down, your heart opens and you share your feelings. At least that's what happens with me. I would like to go on a walk and talk with you—showing you the ExSEPshNL Formula the Lord has shown me. As I show you the exceptional road and the steps that lead to health and well-being. This road is not perfect. It will have bumps and hills and roadblocks, but you won't be alone. I'll be right here with you talking as we go. I'll be asking lots of questions and reminding you of the things you may have once known but forgotten.

My definition of exceptional health is a life where I have less stress, feel better, and have more energy to do the things I love to do. It's not the usual, but it is the road the Lord calls us to travel to become who He has created us to be, living in our fullest spiritual, emotional, and physical state.

This road I am going to show you is a choice every step of the way—it's a road of wellness that allows growth and change daily. My prayer is that this book will help you create your own ***exceptional life***. The best part—it's your life, you are in charge. You get to decide how you want to create it.

If your spiritual, emotional, and physical health is not where you would like it to be—if your past is hindering you from doing what you want to do *today*—if you feel that no matter what you do nothing changes; if you have received the "normal" diagnosis and know there has to be more... I want you to know that the ExSEPshNL Formula™ is for you.

I believe following the ExSEPshNL Formula is the foundation for living an exceptional life. Just as Albert Einstein shared with the world one of the greatest formulas—$E=MC^2$—he did not create energy. The energy was always there for us to use, even if we didn't understand how it worked. Albert Einstein just shared the formula—the *how*.

The exceptional life has always been here for us, we may not have seen the roadmap or understood how to follow the path. I believe God gave me the ExSEPshNL Formula so I could live an exceptional life and share with you how you can too. Without exceptional health, it's almost impossible to live out our purpose. I am not saying your health is going to be perfect. I let go of perfection. Exceptional is not perfection, but it will help you regain control of your health by getting off the normal road that leads to disease and help you discover the skills, tools, and techniques that lead you to the most powerful healer and to receive healing from within.

I know from my experience that ExSEPshNL has been a powerful formula to help me achieve my health goals and live out my purpose, and I believe it can help you achieve yours, too. So let's go together and take a walk and talk and see how you can say *hello exceptional* too.

EXSEPSHNL SPELLED OUT

"To learn to read is to light a fire; every syllable that is spelled out is a spark."
~ Victor Hugo

I like to have a plan of where I am going, the direction I am headed. What I love about the ExSEPshNL Formula that the Lord gave me, it's the roadmap that leads me step by step. But, even with a roadmap, you don't know everything that will come your way—you have to trust Him and learn as you go. As we walk and talk, we will stop at each part of the formula as I share what I have learned on my personal journey. Do you see how the SEP stands out between the small x and the small s in ExSEPshNL? God gave me this beautiful picture of what SEP stands for: the holistic you, your Spiritual, Emotional, and Physical being, all three connected make you—YOU!

ExSEPshNL Formula™

Ex: Exits and Exercises we choose daily for exceptional health

S: Spiritual being - our core, our beliefs, our relationship with God and ourselves

E: Emotional being - our emotions and feelings, our connection with others

P: Physical being - our internal/external organs, our actions performed on this earth

s: sleep and rest - essential for repairing and recharging the spirit, mind, and body

h: hydration - essential for keeping organs functioning properly

N: Nutrition - essential to nourish the body for growth, repair, and energy

L: LIFE (L- Living, I- Investing, F- Finances, E- Energy)

Each day we will begin to look at the different areas of our life and begin to make some changes. Remember, there must be action or no change will occur.

But there is more... curious to see if SEP was an actual word I went on a Google scavenger hunt. *Sep is* short for September our 9th month. I found this interesting because when I had prayed and asked the Lord who He created me to be, the exceptional me. He gave me the 9 *Fruits of the Spirit* from Galatians 5. This is the woman and mom I had always wanted to be—one full of love, joy, peace, patience, kindness, goodness, faithfulness, gentleness, and self-control. A *me*—I thought was impossible to *be*. I find the Fruits of the Spirit interesting because each of these attributes is spiritual by nature; emotional in how we feel and physical in the actions we take.

"But the fruit of the Spirit is love, joy, peace, patience, kindness, goodness, faithfulness, gentleness, self-control; against such things there is no law."

GALATIANS 5: 22-23 (NASB)

Then, as I read more, I found out that in Latin and Greek, *sep* means "7" and represents the 7 *Spirits of God* found in Isaiah 11:1-3. I found this to be important because it is here we find wisdom and understanding through the Holy Spirit—God. So often we look everywhere for the answers, but so many of the answers are already inside of us, all we need to do is ask, listen, and follow through.

"Then a shoot will spring from the stem of Jesse, and a branch from his roots will bear fruit. The Spirit of the LORD will rest on Him, the spirit of wisdom and understanding, the spirit of counsel and strength, the spirit of knowledge and the fear of the LORD. And He will delight in the fear of the LORD, and He will not judge by what His eyes see, nor make a decision by what His ears hear..."

ISAIAH 11:1-3(NASB)

Oh, to travel the road with the 7 *Spirits of God* is an exceptional life. But there was more. I found the 7 *Spiritual gifts.* Yes, each of us has gifts. I knew my gift was to teach you what the Lord had given me, to encourage you to take this road with me, and to give you what you needed to take the next step. I was *called* to lead you diligently, and to show you mercy when you find yourself on the "normal" road, and to smile and wave cheerfully as I pray for you to join me.

"We have different gifts, according to the grace given to each of us. If your gift is prophesying, then prophesy in accordance with your faith; if it is serving, then serve; if it is teaching, then teach; if it is to encourage, then give encouragement; if it is giving, then give generously; if it is to lead, do it diligently; if it is to show mercy, do it cheerfully."
ROMANS 12:6-8 (NIV)

This led me to the Greek word *Septuagint*[1], which is the earliest Greek Bible and often translated as "70." How many times are we asked to forgive? In Matthew, Jesus says we should forgive each other "seventy times seven times."[2]

Then I came to this definition of *sep:* "to touch, bind, join," in plain English defined as "to serve."[3] This is when God showed me when your spiritual, emotional, and physical being is all joined and balanced—you are the whole YOU—you God created to have holistic health. One who has love, joy, peace, patience, kindness, goodness, faithfulness, gentleness, self-control, wisdom, understanding, counsel, strength, knowledge, forgives self and others, and uses the gifts God has given to serve the world.

I believe that our spiritual being is where our beliefs are, and I will share about the heart and the Belief Circle in Chapter 7. The Bible is also a wonderful resource to learn more about our emotions. God shows us it's not the emotion itself that causes us problems, it's the inability to handle our emotions the way God has instructed us that is the issue. Our emotions are (sep) tied to our physical body and often the cause of our physical symptoms. Remember all three together, make YOU! When you look at the ExSEPshNL Formula, I want you to pay special attention to that SEP in the middle. I want you to pay attention to YOU.

In the past ten years, what I have learned on my exceptional health journey more than anything is taking the time to ask questions. With each letter in the formula, I asked questions, and the Lord opened doors.

There is so much we can learn from asking questions, and when we look at our health issues, our circumstances, and our problems from all aspects spiritual, emotional, and physical, we will find the answers are inside of us connected to all three.

THE ESSENTIALS TO LIVING A HEALTHY LIFESTYLE

"Many things are good, many are important, but only a few are essential."
~ D. Todd Christofferson

The ExSEPshNL Formula is the essential equation for living a healthy holistic lifestyle. I agree with the research showing 80 percent of today's diseases are preventable.[4] Walking the normal road leads to spiritual, emotional, and physical imbalance also known as dis-ease. When we follow the ExSEPshNL Formula, we exit the superhighway of normal and we take (or choose) the exceptional road; the one that leads to balance, wholeness, and holistic health. The ExSEPshNL Formula does not have a 100 percent guarantee—remember that you have a past and the other 20 percent[5] of the equation. But the exceptional road can help you appreciate the ever-changing dynamic dance of life that brings you less stress, feeling better and more energy no matter where you are today.

In the following chapters, I share what I have learned in each of these areas. I warn you though, *change* is part of the equation. If you are interested in everything staying the same, you and everything around you, and the word *CHANGE* is a dirty word in your personal dictionary, I understand. Change has been difficult for me, too. In 2018, I even chose the word *change* as my word for the year. My daughter thought I was crazy, but I knew if I continued to let the word—the thought of something new and different coming into my life scare me, then everything would stay the same. The one thing that scares me more than change—*NORMAL*.

"If you will change, everything will change for you.
Don't wait for things to change.
Change doesn't start out there,
change starts within...
All change starts with you."
~ Jim Rohn

I love Jim Rohn quotes, but this one reminds me that so often we want different results in our health, our relationships, our careers, our finances, yet we want to stay the same. It's like we think it's everything but us in this world that is the cause—we want to blame God, our spouse, our kids, neighbors, government, or proclaim that the Universe is against us, but we don't want to take responsibility for our own choices. It's time to write a new chapter in your story—one of change—transformation—beauty out of the ashes. *Ready?*

At the beginning of the book, I gave you a Challenge—to write your vision, your dreams, your goals. If you completed it take time now to read over it. Is this what you want your future story to look like? Make any changes or additions to your story now.

If you did not complete it the first time, no worries. Here is your chance to put change into action. A roadmap only works if you know where you are and where you want to go. When you write your future story, the ExSEPshNL Formula works much like a GPS. When you don't know what you want and where you want to go—you are on the "normal" road—going wherever the world leads you.

> Go to www.shawnacale.com/book-bonus
> **Printable Journal Pages and Bonus Resources**
> **to Live an Exceptional Life.**

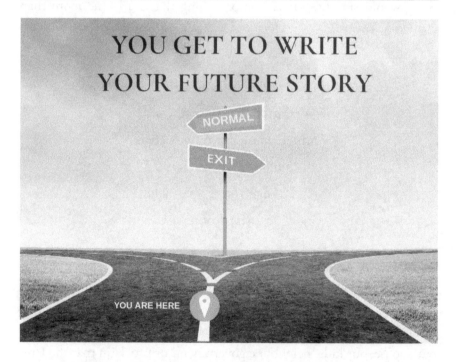

ACTION: WRITE YOUR FUTURE STORY

6

⟨❀⟩

The Ex-It Plan

"For I know the plans I have for you," declares the LORD,
"plans to prosper you and not to harm you,
plans to give you hope and a future."
~ Jeremiah 29:11 (NIV)

The ExSEPshNL Formula starts with Ex and will be our first stop as we walk the exceptional road. My belief was "Ex" must be for exercise. I am a physical therapist and I had spent years instructing my patient's exercises to build up strength and endurance to reach their health goals. I thought the answer to most health problems was exercise. Was the Lord showing me I just needed to exercise more and I would feel better, it would heal me—inside and out? I asked what type of exercises. I started walking again, doing my daily Pilates exercise program, added in strength training as my energy increased. But, as I walked down the road, God showed me "Ex" was much more than exercise. He showed me an Ex-it plan.

> Exit: A way out, a door, to leave, to depart, an outcome.

THE NORMAL ROAD

"Normal is not something to aspire to, it's something to get away from."
~ Jodie Foster

We are habitual human beings. According to the National Science Foundation, we have between 12,000 to 60,000 thoughts per day. I am sure mine is closer to the 60,000. My brain rarely stops. Research shows 95 percent of those thoughts are the same every day. *Guess how many of those thoughts are negative?* 80 percent or more. Wow! Not only are we creatures of habit, but we are also Negative Nellies, too. That's why so many people are on the same road headed in the same direction. It's a comfortable and more traveled road—what I call the "normal" road—and is what leads Americans to the same destination: dis-ease.

Overweight is now the "norm" and 1 in 3 women are now obese. Those over the age of 45 have more than a 50 percent chance of having heart disease. As a woman, you now have a 1 in 2 chance of having cancer in your lifetime. Insulin resistance, pre-diabetes, and diabetes—1 out of 3 people, and 60 percent of people don't even know they have any of the three. After the age of 85, your chance is greater to have Alzheimer's than not. Anxiety and depression are two of the top causes of suicide today and the second leading cause of death among people aged 10-34 years. I know we don't want to hear this. But, if you are traveling the "normal" road, that is where you're headed. That was the road I traveled for almost 40 years. Now, you may think what I thought ten years ago. *What other choice do I have?* Let me tell you, there is hope.

Being overweight, having Alzheimer's, anxiety, cancer, diabetes, depression, and heart disease are all lifestyle diseases, meaning that when you change your lifestyle, you decrease your chance of having any of these diseases. It's pretty empowering if you think about it. Exceptional health is a lifestyle where you focus on holistic health rather than focusing on illness and disease, and when you get off the "normal" road you have much more control over your health.

EX-IT PLAN #1

*"Ninety-nine percent of the failures come from people
who have the habit of making excuses."*
~ George Washington Carver

I believe the number one disease that inflicts us in today's society is not inflammation, obesity, diabetes, heart attacks... while these may cause death, I believe they result from a bigger epidemic—excusitis.

Excusitis: *the inflamed verbiage a person uses to excuse their lack of action and poor results*

Excuse: *(1) an explanation to defend or justify a poor choice (2) a poor example to others*

We can find this disease in most *homo sapiens* (human beings) and spreads rapidly. This is a disease of the mind and symptoms include the normal response to a situation: "If only..."

"If only I were not fat."
"If only I was smarter."
"If only I were healthier."
"If only I had more time."
"If only I were beautiful."
"If only I had a better job."
"If only I had more money."

If only... if only... and it goes on and on.

Unlike most diseases, this one has a cure. Taking responsibility for one's own life. I am going to tell you something I was told a long time ago. The "story" you tell is the story you get. What story (words) is coming out of your mouth? *"Life is too hard."* ~ *"I don't have time to exercise."* ~ *"Losing weight is hard for me."* ~ *"I'm just not consistent enough."* ~ *"We are too busy to eat healthy." ~ "My spouse and kids don't like healthy food." ~ "I don't have the money to eat healthy food."*

I hear myself speak these words and they become my truth. What I think then becomes my story. The more excuses, the more of the same story I create. But when I hear those words come out of someone else's mouth, Wow! They sure have a lot of excuses. Why is it always easier to see the disease in someone else, but we can't see it in ourselves? It's because we wrote our story, we are living our story, and we believe our story. When you can see you are traveling down the road of excuses, you can Ex-it that road and choose a new road, a new story.

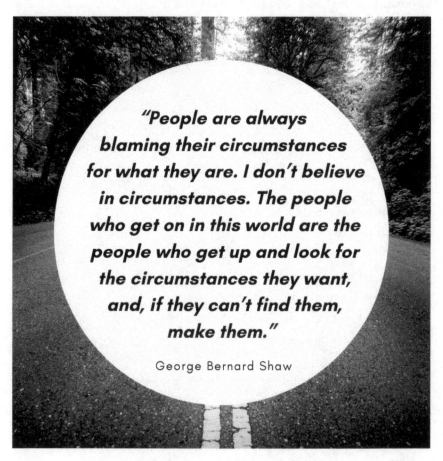

"People are always blaming their circumstances for what they are. I don't believe in circumstances. The people who get on in this world are the people who get up and look for the circumstances they want, and, if they can't find them, make them."

George Bernard Shaw

Where has the road you have been taking led you?
Ready to get off that road?

ANOTHER ROAD

"A dead end can never be a one-way street;
you can always turn around and take another road."
～ Robert Foster Bennett

I shared my story with you for several reasons: one is if you looked at my circumstances and my story, I could have taken another road and not be where I am today; letting my circumstances dictate who I am.

A few years ago, I walked the streets of San Diego and saw young girls sleeping on the side of the road. My heart hurt. I broke down crying as my husband and I walked back to our hotel. My thoughts—what if it had been me?

I've heard, "That would have never been you." But I know the dark road I was traveling. If I had not left the road I was on at 10, I would be in a different place. I often wonder why the girl lying on the hard cement didn't make it out. Why didn't she take an Ex-it? What was different? Why her and not me? I prayed for each girl to realize she could get up and turn around and take another road.

This past year we went to Las Vegas and only after minutes of walking the strip my head ached and my heart grieved. I began feeling the same way I had in San Diego. Maybe even worse, because it seemed as if it was just "normal" to walk down the street and see calling cards of girls selling their bodies—older women with small children passing out the cards to whoever would take them. My heart-broken thinking many of these women believed that's all they deserved; they were not worthy of more. Others in search of love and a sense of value found themselves in this place, not realizing they are victims of sex trafficking.

How many women today do not feel worthy and are traveling the "normal" road? Why is it the average American believes the "normal" road is as good as it gets? What is stopping us from living the exceptional life… a life of holistic health?

Every day, I have the choice of how I am going to write my story, *"I don't have time to take care of myself,"* or *"I have time every day to take care of myself because I am worth it."*

The girls and women who are slaves and do not have the choice, or those who do not realize other choices exist, need us. These women need us to be strong. We must become healthy enough to find them, see them, help them, support them on their road to recovery.

As you write your new story to reflect your desires, your dreams, you will see a change in yourself and in your life. You will also have those moments when you argue with yourself and say, "No, I don't have time to exercise; I need to ..." I have found arguing with myself doesn't work. There is never a clear winner. What I have found works: asking myself questions regarding the road I am traveling.

> *Why don't I have time to exercise today?*
> *Do I have too many things on my plate?*
> *What could I change so I have time to exercise today?*
> *Could I mark off time on my calendar so I don't fill it up?*

Often, I find I have time. I was making an excuse, also known as a well-planned lie, going back to my old story, listening to the lies. I recognize we live in a microwave world. We want instant change; instant results. But we are not a microwave, we are complex; we are human. Change takes time. Every one of our 100 trillion cells has heard the same story over and over. Until our cells hear the new story and our inner self believes it, our self will want to return to what it knows; that's why we call it a *habit*. We may find ourselves every morning back on the normal road, but we get to choose the road we take.

What excuses have you been speaking?
What circumstances have been stopping you?
Are you ready to go down a new road?

A MIRACLE

"Do you want to get well?"
~ John 5:6b (NIV)

Perhaps, like me, you have prayed and searched for a miracle. Did you know in the Bible each miracle occurred when someone in the story was *called* to do something? In John chapter 5, a man had been lame for 38 years when Jesus asked him, *"Do you want to get well?"* The man did not answer with a "Yes!" Instead, the invalid replied, *"Sir, I have no one to help me into the pool when the water is stirred. While I am trying to get in, someone else goes down ahead of me."* Could these have been excuses? *"Then Jesus said to him, 'Get up! Pick up your mat and walk.' At once the man picked up his mat and walked."*

When I read this story with fresh eyes from this perspective, I remembered when I was 38 years old going through my health crisis and going from doctor to doctor looking for answers, but I wasn't doing the things I knew to do for my health—like this man I was making excuses yet asking for a miracle.

When God gave me the ExSEPshNL Formula, I felt He was saying STOP the excuses and the old habits blocking you from living an exceptional life. He gave me the action plan I needed to receive my personal miracle. I just had to get up and walk. Why are we afraid to pick up our mat and walk? Is it out of fear of failure? I can only imagine how this man who had been an invalid for 38 years felt. *It's impossible, I will make a fool of myself. This is just the way I am.* It says, "he was cured." I wonder what he was cured of? Maybe he had the disease—excusitis and when he picked up his mat and walked the excuses fell off.

I have met no one who has said, "I want to be unhealthy." I have met and worked with hundreds of people who, when I gave them instructions to help them get better, had more than a few excuses for why they couldn't do the things they needed to do to become healthy. Excuses seem to stop us before we ever get started. Just like Jesus in this passage, I am going to challenge you to pick up your mat and walk.

**Go to www.shawnacale.com/book-bonus
Printable Journal Pages and Bonus Resources
to Live an Exceptional Life.**

ACTION: EXIT THE "NORMAL" ROAD OF EXCUSES

1. Write on a piece of paper or in your journal the excuses blocking you from reaching your goals.

2. Write what lies you have been believing and how they have affected your health.

3. Write one action you already know you can do today to feel better tomorrow.

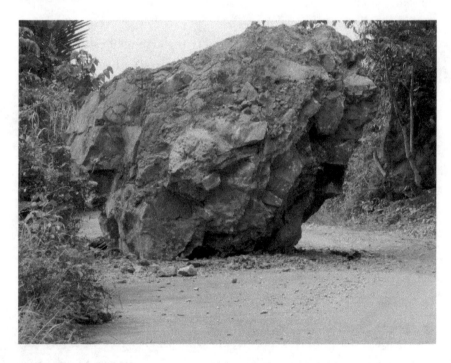

Ex-It Plan #1: Exit the Normal Road of Excuses.

EX-IT! PLAN #2

"In everything set them an example by doing what is good."
~ Titus 2:7 (NIV)

I know taking the "normal" road seems easier. Walk with me. Let me show you another way, another Ex-it. Remember definition number 2 of *excuse: "a poor example to others."*

When we Ex-It off the *Excuse Road* we can take the *Be An Example Road*. I don't know about you, but as a woman, Christ-follower, wife, mom, daughter, sister, friend, leader and the list goes on, I want to be a positive example. I don't want to take someone down a road that leads to pain or disease.

People are watching you. Whether you want them to—they see you; they hear you; they learn from you. What is it they see, hear, and learn?

When I thought about my daughter and my sons and how they were watching the choices I was making, I knew I did not want them to make those same choices. I looked more closely at the road I was traveling. When I said, I was too busy to go for a walk, but had time to watch a TV show; what type of example was I showing them? When I checked my emails and/or social media before spending time in the Word, what type of example was I showing my family on what was most important to me—God or the world? When I yelled and would get angry for minor mistakes my children would make, what type of example was I setting for them now and as they become parents, too? When I would choose sugar and products like a white flour tortilla after already learning the power these two have over my system, what type of example am I setting? When I travel the "normal" road—the road that often feels like the easier road to take, the one that everyone else is going down, the one that has advertisements and billboards pointing in the direction to go every day—I have to ask myself, *Is this the road I want to take my family, friends and everyone else down?* Or do I want to be an example—the one who takes the exit off the normal road and leads the way for others to see there is another way—an exceptional way?

Go to www.shawnacale.com/book-bonus
Printable Journal Pages and Bonus Resources
to Live an Exceptional Life.

ACTION: TAKE THE BE AN EXAMPLE ROAD

1. Write on a piece of paper or in your journal the people you want to set an example for in your life.

2. How could you encourage others by being an example.

3. Write one action you can do today to be an example to someone in your life.

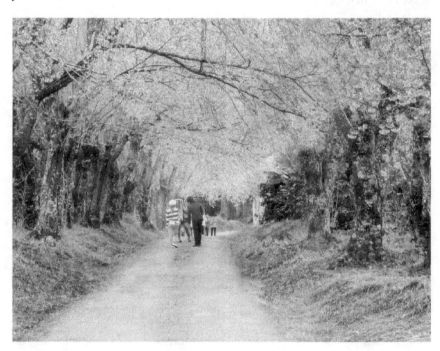

Ex-It Plan #2: Be an Example.

EX-IT PLAN #3

"The body heals with play, the mind heals with laughter,
and the spirit heals with joy."
~ Proverb

As we exit off the road of excuses and onto the be an example road, it's time to set our GPS with some coordinates. I have found Ex-It #3 is exercise, and each one I set in my GPS strengthens me and my health.

Often, when we hear the word *exercise*, we think only about exercising our body and we think it's difficult, time-consuming and the word itself may even make you feel overwhelmed. Remember we are spiritual, emotional, and physical beings, and the word *exercise* is a term used to bring growth in all areas.

EXERCISE
(1) activity requiring physical effort to sustain or improve health
(2) a process or activity carried out for a specific purpose
(3) to improve a specific area or skill in life

Each letter in the ExSEPshNL Formula represents an area we must take responsibility for in our life for exceptional health. Ex comes first so we can exercise in all areas to have holistic health. I have found that if I have an Ex-it (exercise—micro-commitment, an activity to improve health for each area) I grow spiritually, emotionally, and physically. I become self-disciplined, resilient, and strong.

ExSEPshNL Solution: Take Responsibility for Your Life

TREE ANALOGY

*"We are like the little branch that quivers during a storm,
doubting our strength and forgetting we are the tree—
deeply rooted to withstand all life's upheavals."*
~ Dodinsky

As we walk together, let's look at the trees. See the big, tall trees with the vast root system and wide trunks, they are strong and produce many leaves and much fruit. See the small trees with little to no root systems they can handle very little and have a hard time producing any fruit. Have you ever noticed throughout scripture trees are used to represent humans?

> *"That person is like a tree planted by streams of water, which yields its fruit in season and whose leaf does not wither— whatever they do prospers."*
>
> PSALM 1:3 (NIV)

Did you know trees grow stronger and more resilient with the stress of the wind, storms, drought, and other elements? How do they handle it all? It all starts with having a strong root system. As tree roots grow deeper their trunk grows wider. The bigger the trunk, the more the tree can handle. Do you know what a healthy tree produces? Fruit. I want you to think of the exercises we will talk about as ways to grow your roots deeper, stronger, and towards the water.

Roots to me look like different roads that all lead to the trunk. I have found all the areas in the ExSEPshNL Formula are part of the root system, and each area has a specific purpose in having exceptional health and living an exceptional life.

When you perform each exercise, a micro-commitment towards living an exceptional life, you are practicing self-discipline. The more self-discipline, the easier it is to follow through with your commitments. This is a two-way road that leads you to an exceptional life.

When I picture living an exceptional life, I see myself as a beautiful rainbow eucalyptus tree. If you have never seen one it is unusual, not typical, and I would call it outstanding—it's considered a little messy, large and takes up space with deep widespread roots. I imagine the fruit (gumnuts) on my tree being the nine fruits of the spirit.

Would you like to have more of the fruit of self-discipline?
If you were more self-disciplined, would it be easier to be healthy?

Go to www.shawnacale.com/book-bonus
Printable Journal Pages and Bonus Resources
to Live an Exceptional Life.

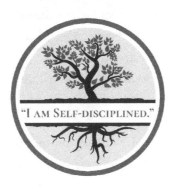

"I AM SELF-DISCIPLINED."

ACTION: EXERCISE

1. Write on a piece of paper or in your journal some areas in your life where self-discipline could help you become healthier.

2. What is one exercise (small micro-commitment) you could begin today to live a healthier lifestyle?

Ex-It Plan #3: Exercise

THE MAGIC PILL

"A little magic can take you a long way."
~ Roald Dahl

If I knew about a little "magic pill" that could help you be more self-disciplined, feel and look younger, lowered stress, reduced the risk of heart disease, improved blood pressure, lowered the risk of obesity, increased energy, and enhanced well-being would you want me to share it with you?

What if this "magic pill" didn't cost you an extra penny?

Only 20 percent of the American population exercise daily. The other 80 percent are part of the "norm"—the ones who do not exercise—this pill is for you. Now to get this "magic pill" for free you must go out each day to get it, it's about a 15-minute walk away from any location you start. That's part of the magic. Once you get there, you walk 15 minutes back to your destination. Simple. No shortcuts.

Did you figure out the magic part? Studies show "one" type of exercise works better than any actual "pill" they have put it up against. Walking.[1]

As a physical therapist, I would often tell my patients, "If you don't use it you will lose it." That includes walking. Want to walk for the rest of your life and do the things you want to do? Walking will get you there. I can't tell you how many times I worked with patients who hadn't walked over 200 feet in their homes for months, even years. They lost the ability. They would come to the hospital scared to take a step. The doctor would often tell me they could go home when they could walk 500 feet. It felt impossible to them, but I knew that if I could help them take that first step, the fear would begin to disappear and they could take another and then another, and with time and strengthening they would reach their goal—they would return home.

I believe most people KNOW they NEED to walk or do some physical exercise daily. My question is WHY are only 20 percent of Americans doing it?

Realistically, the other 80 percent have excusitis. Let's go over the top 10 excuses and find a few solutions (exits) to help you take that First Step.

TOP 10 EXCUSES NOT TO WALK

Excuse #1: *Not enough time.* The recommended amount of walking per week is 150 minutes or 30 minutes per day, five days a week.

Solution: The average American watches 4.3 hours of TV a day. Turn off the TV and put in your earbuds and walk 30 minutes instead.

Excuse #2: *Too busy.* You have work, school, cooking, cleaning, shopping, kids, laundry... the list goes on and on. There isn't enough time to do everything. Studies show that Americans are working less per day than they were 10 years ago, yet we are busier.

Solution: Planning sessions and self-discipline are a great way to let go of busyness. Schedule walking like you do every other important appointment. You are worth it!

Excuse #3: *I don't want to walk alone.* Many people are afraid to walk alone.

Solution: Find a walking partner. Whether it is a family member (bonding time), a neighbor, friend, or maybe it's time to get a dog. Don't let this excuse stop you from walking. There are walking groups and walking clubs that often gather at local parks and malls. Maybe it's time to join one.

Excuse #4: Weather. *It's too hot, it's too cold, it's raining, it's windy, it's...*

Solution: You can walk inside a mall. Going to the grocery store? Walk around the parameter several times before you grab that shopping cart. It might surprise you how much walking you can get done in your own home. Walk through the entire house several times. Be creative.

Excuse #5: *I'm too tired.* Most people with this excuse are tired because they sit for a living.

Solution: Getting up and moving will increase blood circulation and before you know it you have more energy. Energy begets energy.

Excuse #6: I'm sore. My legs hurt, my feet hurt, my...

Solution: Unless you have an injury, don't stop walking. Your body is getting stronger and your muscles are getting accustomed to it. A nice Epsom Salt bath with essential oils or soaking your feet will help relieve some soreness.

Excuse #7: *I'm out of shape.* Getting started doesn't mean you have to walk a mile or a 5k.

Solution: Start slow. If 10 minutes is all you can handle, then walk that amount every day for a week. Then add another 10-minute session until you can walk 10 minutes three times a day. Then increase your time to 20 minutes and work your way to 30 minutes.

Excuse #8: Unmotivated. *I know I need to, but I just can't make myself do it.*

Solution: Sometimes we need something external to motivate us internally. Maybe a fresh pair of walking shoes or a new walking outfit. Maybe one of the cool fitness trackers that measures your steps and/or distance. Are you motivated by a challenge? Sign up for a walking challenge.

Excuse #9: *Walking is boring.* Americans are used to being entertained. We watch TV; we get on our computers, smartphones, and watch what everyone else is doing. Then we go on a walk and find it boring.

Solution: Find a beautiful place around a pond, lake, or fountain to do your daily walk. If entertainment motivates, put in your earbuds and listen to a book, podcast, or your favorite music. Need more visual input? Walk on a treadmill in front of a television during your favorite show.

Excuse #10: *I just don't like to exercise.* Often, this is just the plain truth. Some people just don't like to move; they prefer to be static.

Solution: Sometimes we have to do the things we don't like to live the life we want. Do you want to walk around the store to buy your own groceries? Do you want to walk to the sports field to watch your grandchildren play ball? Do you want to live a life of health and wellness? Then the solution is to get up and walk.

Hippocrates said, "Walking is man's best medicine"
and thousands of years later, the results are in—he was right!

FIRST STEP

We know exercise is part of living a more holistic lifestyle. Walking is one of the most underrated exercise options. We often make things more difficult than they have to be. Study after study has shown that walking is the easiest, cheapest, most functional, and beneficial exercise that we can do daily. Research has proven that something as simple as walking can prevent disease, yet we keep looking for more answers and we haven't even taken the first step.

What if...

walking 30 minutes a day prevented you from a heart attack or stroke?
walking prevented you from having diabetes or high blood pressure?
walking daily allowed you to live a long life with those you love?

Making healthy choices such as walking daily may not always be easy, but for every excuse, we can find a solution. Walking is not just a physical exercise; there has been proof that it helps our spiritual and emotional health, too.[2] A simple way is to turn your walk into a prayer and/or gratitude walk.[3] When we add prayer to our walk, we gain the spiritual connection that many of us are looking for and add in gratitude, the greatest cure for a broken heart and you're on your healthy way.

> *"Gratitude is the closest thing you have to a cure-all 'magic elixir' for anything life may throw at you."*
> ~Unknown

Focusing on gratitude gives you strength, allows you to see from a new perspective, it replaces worry, and puts less stress on your heart. It allows you to move forward while letting go of the things stopping you. I have spent seasons of my life taking prayer walks as I talk to God and build a relationship with Him. I talk to Him about my fears and I pray for those I love. I also spend time on my walks finding all the things I am grateful for, and my youngest son Bryce and I have played the Gratitude game on our walk and talks. I say something I am grateful for and then he does the same. It often starts with being grateful for one another and moves to being grateful for the trees, the grass, the pond, the ducks, the sun, the cool wind, the sound of the leaves rustling. But with time as we continue, we become grateful for the hard things.

Research shows those who do gratitude walks are happier people. Going for a gratitude walk any time of the day is a good time, but first thing in the morning starts your day exceptionally. Remember, 30 minutes is only 1/24th of your day. Giving you 23 1/2 hours to do everything else.

> *It's not happiness that brings us gratitude.*
> *It's gratitude that brings us happiness.*
> ~Anonymous

Go to www.shawnacale.com/book-bonus
Printable Journal Pages and Bonus Resources
to Live an Exceptional Life.

EXERCISE: WALK

1. Are you part of the 80 or 20 percent regarding daily exercise?

2. What would a life of self-discipline, prayer/gratitude and a daily walk do for you?

3. Commit to Take the First Step of the ExSEPshNL Formula—Walk. Share your commitment with someone to keep you accountable.

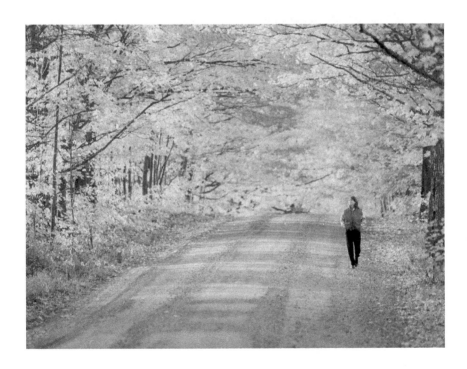

ExSEPshNL Formula: First Step—Walk

7

The Spiritual Core

"If we don't build our Spiritual core our world is going to collapse."
~ Christine Caine

As we continue our walk and talk, our next stop in the ExSEPshNL Formula is the "S" for Spiritual health—our core, our beliefs, our relationship with God, and ourselves. This is the topic I argued with God, yes God, at the beginning about why I could not write this book. I think this topic scared me more than any other topic to write about—fear that I wouldn't write the right thing. The pressure of what other Christians would think. Opinions of what non-Christians believe. Just the *thought* stopped me in my tracks.

Have you ever thought about where your thoughts come from or the fact they lead you on the road you are traveling down? The funny thing is this one word—*thought*—led me on an unexpected journey that has brought me more light, more answers, and, most of all, something I am very passionate to share with you today.

> Thought: An idea or opinion produced by thinking.

When I prayed to God to show me what *spiritual health* meant and how to grow in this area, He again used the tree analogy to help me visualize our spiritual being and how it plays a part in our holistic health. He showed me the inside of a tree—specifically the rings you see when you cut down a tree. In the center you see this beautiful darker core—it's very apparent in a cedarwood tree. The bigger the center core, the stronger the tree. I call this the SEP Circle—YOU.

The cedarwood tree kept coming back to me, so I looked up what it means. *It is a symbol of antiquity, immensity, and enduring strength... symbolic meanings of healing, cleansing, rituals of protection, resilience, support, strength, and hope.*[2]

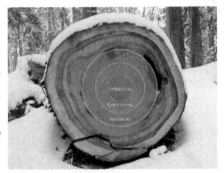

I don't know about you, but those qualities all sound wonderful to have as a human, too.

Like a tree that grows fruit, it must have deep roots and a sturdy trunk and water to promote growth. This is where the spiritual fruits in Galatians Chapter 5 came into the picture the Lord gave me. I pictured the core of the tree to be our heart, what many consider our spiritual center, and I believe that which connects our spiritual being, emotional being, and physical being all into one—SEP. This then led me to love—not just any love—unconditional love. But now I am jumping to the end of the chapter; and I want to take you back to that word: *thought*.

ExSEPshNL Solution: Unconditional Love

BELIEF CIRCLE

"As he thinks in his heart, so is he."
~ Proverbs. 23:7 (NKJV)

I read a lot of books and I am not sure if one specific book or a few of them together brought me my interpretation of the Belief Circle. I believe we hold our beliefs in our spiritual core—the heart. Within our core belief system comes our thoughts and from our thoughts, our emotions, and from our emotions, our feelings, and from our feelings come our actions and from our actions, we see our results and that leads us back to proving or disproving our beliefs and the circle continues.

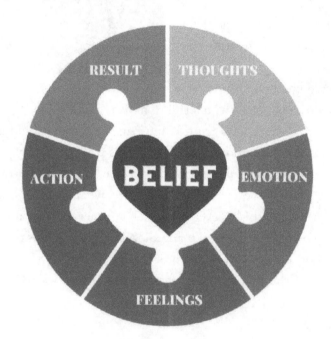

Now let's go back to my *thought* when I heard the Lord speak to me about writing this book. "What will people think about a Christian using the word *spiritual?*"

Where did that *thought* come from? Did it just appear out of thin air and into my brain? I think not. I somehow had formed a belief from what I had heard, read, or from someone that I trusted—*Christians dislike the word spiritual.* The more I think about it, the crazier it sounds, but that's what I believed. That *thought* brought up an emotion, and the emotion was fear. Many say that all emotions stem from either love or fear, and everything I was feeling was coming from the fear side. This led me to feel as though I could not write this book, which stopped me from publishing this book for almost 10 years. My result—10 years of excuses and disobedience to the Lord—blocking me from fully living my exceptional life. What changed? My belief.

When I was writing my story over and over through my healing process, I saw beliefs popping up here and there. I questioned why I believed what I believe. Let me tell you, questioning your own beliefs is difficult—what you believe is your truth. Most of us will fight for our beliefs because it's what we stand for. But what if your belief is not the truth? *Then what?* This is where I found myself multiple times over the years. What did I find? When I questioned my beliefs—my truths, I had breakthroughs, growth in myself, and in my health. I want this for you too. I want you to look over your story and see what beliefs have been moving you forward and giving you the results you desire and what beliefs have been stopping you from fulfilling who God created you to be.

Have you set a goal and found yourself not meeting it?
Could it be your beliefs—your truth—in conflict with your goal?

EMPOWERING BELIEFS

"The real challenge is to choose, hold, and operate through intelligent, uplifting, and fully empowering beliefs."
~ Michael Sky

In the first six years of our life, we create most of our core beliefs. Each belief formed from our experiences (the outside world) and our personal viewpoint (personality). As we have new experiences and new input coming in through our senses—touch, sight, hearing, smell, and taste—a belief is born. When reading the *"heads"* side of my penny story—you can find empowering beliefs scattered throughout.

"I am loved."

"I am special."

"I am happy."

"I am adventurous."

"I love to learn."

"I help women."

Every one of those empowering beliefs has led me to thoughts of "I can". Bringing me emotions from the love side and feelings of joy and happiness. These feelings led me to take actions such as going to college, getting married, having children, traveling to far-off places, studying and researching, having fun, and helping women feel better. Without empowering beliefs, I could not have accomplished what I have accomplished with the successful results I have had in my life.

You too have accomplished amazing things
because of your empowering beliefs.

LIMITING BELIEFS

"The only thing limiting you is yourself."
~ Ken Poirot

As we grow, we keep our old beliefs, or we can create new beliefs. Yes, we create new beliefs as time goes by from our experiences, and even from our thought life. We can even change our beliefs. Remember, every penny has a *"tails"* side too—and the flip side is our limiting beliefs. Throughout my story, I could also see the limiting beliefs that stopped, blocked, and prevented me from living out my full potential. Often, trauma or unexpected results can form a new belief or even flip an empowering belief to a limiting belief.

As I looked over the *"tails"* side of my story, I saw so many limiting beliefs.

"I am a mistake."

"I am special."

"I am pretty."

"I am bad."

"I am not good enough."

"I am not worthy."

You might say, "Wait, Shawna, you have some empowering beliefs mixed in with limiting beliefs. How can that be?" Great question and an eye-opening experience for me, for sure. God showed me this clear picture when my oldest son Ryan and daughter Emily were studying the book of James many years ago. I was double-minded in so many areas of my life, and it was all rooted in my core beliefs. Don't worry. I will unfold more of this as we go, but for now, let's move on to the truth.

"A double minded man is unstable in all his ways."

JAMES 1:8 (KJV)

**What limiting beliefs are blocking you
from the exceptional life, you desire?**

TRUTH

"Most people argue over beliefs rather than truth."
~ S.C. Meaken

Truth: What is it? The *Oxford English Dictionary* says *a fact or belief that is accepted as true.* But what happens when my belief differs from your belief? Which one is true? Well, let's be honest: We are always going to vote for our own belief—it is our truth. That's why we have war, fighting, disagreements, and arguments... because we don't all believe the same thing. We ALL have had unique experiences and have seen those through different lenses. This was hard for me because I see through the lenses of right and wrong and my belief was, "I am always right." I say "was" because I have learned I must test my beliefs.

So how do we test our beliefs? There are several ways. First, as a Christian, I can test my beliefs against the Word of God. Second, I have learned to test my beliefs against my thoughts, my emotions, my feelings, my actions, and my results. We often say, "I believe..." but we spend the day 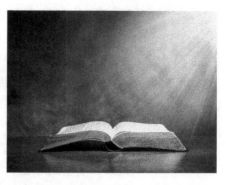 thinking about something different. If we truly believed what we said, why would we not spend our time thinking about it? Or we say, "I believe everything will be fine" yet we are worried and stressed regarding the very thing we say we are fine about. How often do you say, "I know I need to..." yet you don't do it? Could it be a limiting belief? What if we say, "I believe..." but our results do not show that belief in action? Is there another belief overriding that one?

Without truth, it is very difficult for our whole-self to stay in harmony. Our truth leads us down the road we are traveling. I have found when our beliefs are rooted in truth, we find freedom.

THOUGHTS

"Change your thoughts and you change your world."
~ Norman Vincent Peale

I remember my darkest days and the thoughts ruminating in my head. I also remember my happiest days and the thoughts I would meditate upon. Why did it take so long to realize what I thought affected my emotions? You may believe *I cannot control my thoughts, my emotions, or how I feel.* Oh, how I get you! I thought like this for so many years. I remember when my emotions would roar and I would think, *This is just who I am and if you don't like it, get out of the way, because that means you don't like me.*

Okay, now as I read the words, I can see how my pastor could see the hostility within me. There is only so much of ourselves we can hide, and our thoughts will show either by the words we speak, our facial expressions, body language, or overall disposition. If it's possible to change our thoughts—how do we?

CHOICE

"Today I have given you the choice between life and death,
between blessings and curses. Now I call on heaven and earth
to witness the choice you make. Oh, that you would choose life,
so that you and your descendants might live!"
~ Deuteronomy 30:19 (NLT)

Choice. *Could it be that easy?* For years I would read Deuteronomy 30:19 and think I don't have control over whether I live or die. Until... that moment in the ambulance. Sure, I needed the help of the paramedic and the doctor, but I believe the moment I made the choice to live—things changed. I had spent so much time thinking (thoughts) that I wasn't enough for my family and going down this spiral of all I had to do to be worthy. It was exhausting. At the end of Chapter 2, I shared this thought: *"I am a failure—failure as a wife, as a mom, as a human being. I am not worthy to live."*

What type of curses had I placed on myself? How was what I was thinking about affecting my health, my life? *Why was I not choosing life?* Do our thoughts play that BIG of a role in our health?

In the early days of my journey, around 2013, I read the book *Who Switched Off My Brain?*[3], by Dr. Caroline Leaf and then a few years later her book *Switch On Your Brain*[4] I enjoyed reading how a communication pathologist, cognitive neuroscientist, brought science and scripture together and was proving what we think changes our brain. We can replace toxic thoughts with healthy thoughts. I felt this could be another missing link to my personal health and the health of so many others.

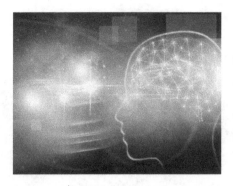

"As we think, we change the physical nature of our brain. As we consciously direct our thinking, we can wire out toxic patterns of thinking and replace them with healthy thoughts."

~Dr. Caroline Leaf

"We demolish arguments and every pretension that sets itself up against the knowledge of God, and we take captive every thought to make it obedient to Christ."

2 CORINTHIANS 10:5 (NIV)

**Go to www.shawnacale.com/book-bonus
Printable Journal Pages and Bonus Resources
to Live an Exceptional Life.**

CHALLENGE: TAKE THOUGHTS CAPTIVE

1. A penny for your thoughts. Today, spend some time taking your thoughts captive and writing them down on paper or in your journal.

2. Would you speak these thoughts out loud upon others? Why or why not?

3. Would you share your thoughts with others? Why or why not?

WORDS

"Gentle words bring life and health; a deceitful tongue crushes the spirit."
~ Proverbs 15:4 (NLT)

Choice. As I captured my thoughts in my journal, I found the words coming from my mouth became more positive. I was now realizing how the words I spoke to my children, my husband, family, and friends affected our relationships. If my words had power, I wanted to use my power for good—I wanted to help moms become healthier. I knew as a woman, the caretaker of the home, we are the example our family sees, hears, and follows. As I dove into the power of words, I learned so much from scripture—the book of Proverbs has dozens of verses on the tongue and the words we speak. The more I studied the Word of God, all the way from the beginning in Genesis when God spoke, *"Let there be light."* I saw the power of the Word in action.

As I continued to pray and ask God more questions, I found the Word of God to have the answers. When reading Psalm 119 I could see what would direct me down the road, I was to take. As I spent more time meditating on the Word, I found my own words changing and saw what I was creating in my life.

"Thy word is a lamp unto my feet, and a light unto my path."
PSALM 119:105 (KJV)

If you are a visual learner like me, you may enjoy the research of Dr. Masaru Emoto. He did amazing experiments on water molecules and found that words altered the molecular structure of water. I have also seen experiments done with rice and how negative words caused the rice to mold sooner than the rice that had positive words spoken over it. Studies have even shown how a plant spoken words of love will thrive, while a plant ignored will shrivel up and die.

What are the words you are speaking about creating in your life?

FLIP THE PENNY PRINCIPLE

"Do not be conformed to this world, but be transformed by the renewal
of your mind, that by testing you may discern what is the will of God,
what is good and acceptable and perfect."
~ Romans 12:2 (ESV)

I was done allowing my limiting beliefs, my negative thoughts, and the words I spoke on myself and others to lead me down the road I was traveling. How do we discern if a core belief is empowering or limiting? As you will see, it's not always a positive against a negative. Just like the penny has two sides, and the tails side isn't the bad guy we can learn from all of our experiences and all of our beliefs. As I tested my beliefs, my thoughts, my words I found my way to exceptional.

I coined the phrase *Flip the Penny Principle*™ when I realized I could flip a limiting belief to an empowering belief, just like I flip a coin. How? I used my thoughts, my words. They are much more powerful than we give them credit. When we form them into "I am..." statements or what many call affirmations, we begin to feel the change.

Let's talk about the belief, "I am special." When I was telling my *"heads"* story—I shared as a little girl I felt special when I received attention. What little girl doesn't want to feel special? When I found out what my grandpa and my neighbor were doing was bad, I had a new thought. But I still had the belief "I am special" and the feeling I liked led to the action—lying—so I could continue to feel special. The results I received were mixed or "double-minded." I believed what they were doing was bad, but the feeling special felt good. As time went on, my feelings matched my thoughts—no longer did I feel good when I went to the neighbor's house. The action changed, and the results changed.

Affirmation: Supporting the value of something, someone, and/or self.

Yet, I had connected the core belief "I am special" with the negative feeling and it became a limiting belief. Whenever I felt "special" the bad feeling would present itself, and I would stop whatever I was doing making me feel special. When I realized this limiting belief, I could use my tools to make changes.

Often, an empowering belief is showing up as a limiting belief when trauma has occurred. The good news is we get to choose our beliefs. I *thought* of times when I felt special with my husband, my kids, friends, those I trusted and connected these feelings with the belief "I am special."

As I continued to grow, I could see how limiting beliefs such as "I am not good enough" was affecting my life and how I could flip it to "I am good enough." Just saying the words "I am good enough" at first was awkward, but with time and practice it felt more natural and, again, empowering. I now use affirmations daily and have found the *Flip the Penny Principle* to be an exceptional tool in my toolbox for life-changing transformation.

If our thoughts come from our beliefs, then choosing our thoughts, re-writing our thoughts, flipping our thoughts is where we can start. A thought that tears down something, someone, or ourselves will never help us reach our goals or our dreams, it will always block our exceptional life. When we can flip that thought to one that builds up, supports, and affirms, this is when we transform our hearts, our minds, our life. The more we go through the belief circle with this new thought and have new experiences, we find that we have flipped our penny and we are living the life we were created to live.

In Chapter 1, I gave you the challenge to write your own Penny Story. Did you do it? If not, no worries, we must be a lot alike. I tend to just keep on reading and learning and not putting things into action, always with the thought, *I'll go back and do it later*.

Flip the Penny Principle: Choosing the side of the coin you want to live by.

Here's the secret I have learned on my long journey: We often make things harder than it needs to be. We may not always understand why we face certain challenges. But when we move through challenges is when we grow. When you do these challenges, I have for you; you grow. Just like we must have empowering thoughts to help us on our journey, we must take that first step of faith and perform the action. If the thoughts of performing a specific action bring up emotions we don't want to feel—like fear, then it is a good sign we have found what is limiting us because fear is what creates limiting beliefs. The flip side is faith, and it shows we are moving in the right direction—one towards growth. Taking the step forward and trusting the process is the beauty of the journey. Whether you did or didn't complete the challenge in Chapter 1, this would be a good time to go back and do it. *Why?* Because when you write your penny story, you will see the limiting beliefs holding you back from reaching true holistic health.

Are you ready to live a life from empowering beliefs?

**Go to www.shawnacale.com/book-bonus
Printable Journal Pages and Bonus Resources
to Live an Exceptional Life.**

ACTION: FLIP THE PENNY™

1. Read over your Penny Story you wrote in Chapter 1 or write your Penny Story now.

2. Find beliefs, often disguised as excuses, that have stopped, blocked, or prevented you from achieving the results you desire? Highlight them and make a list.

3. Write a few affirmations from your list to speak daily.

FLIP THE PENNY PRINCIPLE™

5 SIMPLE STEPS

Your **limiting** beliefs are hiding out in the areas where you're producing results you don't want.

Step 1: Write the **limiting belief** down...

Step 2: Acknowledge these are **beliefs**, not truths!

Step 3: Flip the **belief**...

Step 4: Write an affirmation for your new **empowering belief.**

Step 5: Take different actions to prove the new belief.

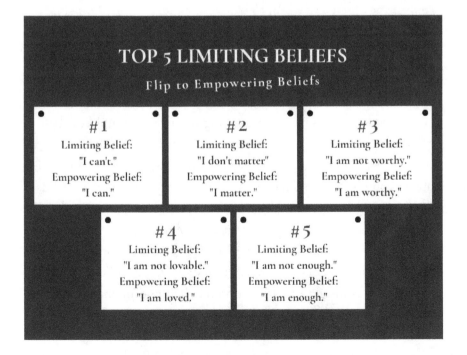

TOP 5 LIMITING BELIEFS

Flip to Empowering Beliefs

#1
Limiting Belief:
"I can't."
Empowering Belief:
"I can."

#2
Limiting Belief:
"I don't matter"
Empowering Belief:
"I matter."

#3
Limiting Belief:
"I am not worthy."
Empowering Belief:
"I am worthy."

#4
Limiting Belief:
"I am not lovable."
Empowering Belief:
"I am loved."

#5
Limiting Belief:
"I am not enough."
Empowering Belief:
"I am enough."

LOVE

"Love is patient, love is kind.
It does not envy, it does not boast, it is not proud.
It does not dishonor others, it is not self-seeking,
it is not easily angered, it keeps no record of wrongs.
Love does not delight in evil but rejoices with the truth.
It always protects, always trusts, always hopes, always perseveres.
Love never fails."
~ 1 Corinthians 13:4-8a (NIV)

Our spiritual core: our beliefs—our heart, our thoughts, our words—all stem from either fear or love. As I was walking this journey and trying to better understand what God was teaching me on the spiritual aspect, I felt as if the fruits of the spirit were key to unlocking the answer to my questions.

"But the fruit of the Spirit is love, joy, peace, patience, kindness,
goodness, faithfulness, gentleness and self-control."
GALATIANS 5:22-23 (NIV)

One late night I was messaging a friend, coach, colleague of sorts about questions I was having pertaining to my beliefs and how best to walk through the process. She asked me to test for love/hate.

Now you may think that to be an odd question, or even question how do you test love and hate? As a physical therapist, for years I used muscle testing to determine a person's muscle strength, but in the past few years, I have learned more about muscle testing and applied kinesiology. There are several kinesiology muscle-testing techniques used to see if a stressor or abnormal nervous system input weakens a muscle. This can give us insight into how certain beliefs and/or emotions are affecting us.

A self-muscle-testing technique I like to use is the *Sway Test*. The premise behind it is we sway (move) forward to the things we desire, a "yes" or a strong and/or positive response, or an empowering belief. We sway backward to the things we do not desire, our "no," or a weak and/or negative response, or a limiting belief.

Now, logically, I am thinking, love would be a positive (forward) sway and hate would be a negative (backward) sway, What I have learned about beliefs is that they are not always logical. I tested myself, interestingly enough, that one question sent me on a week-long quest with lots of prayers, meditating on scriptures, and fasting.

When I tested "hate" it was a negative (backward) sway as expected, but "love" was a negative (backward) sway for me too. How could love—something good—be something I would test weak from? Why would I pull away—fall backward—to that which brings such joy and happiness?

Could it be that love to me was a limiting belief? How does one go through life with love being a negative? I asked myself more questions: "Does Jesus love me?" That was "Yes!" Okay, "Does God love me?" Another forward sway "Yes." I would repeat the word "love" all alone and again I would get a "No." After praying that night and asking God questions for clarity in response to love, I kept hearing the love passage in 1 Corinthians 13. *"Love never fails."*

Those three words kept flowing through my thoughts. If love never fails, then why am I backing away—why am I not running toward love? Then I thought about my story. Do I love myself? I quickly fell backwards. It was a big fat "no." It made complete sense in so many ways. I knew from my own thoughts I needed to love myself more, but I would always put it into the "I need to do more self-care, take more time for myself." But it was so eye-opening to test those words and see that one of my limiting beliefs was I didn't love myself—at least not in the same sense that God loves me.

I dove deeper into the word—*love.* I had put so many conditions on myself that the love I had for myself was just that—*conditional* love. The voices in my head were nagging, "Shawna, to be loved you must do this, do that, do it perfectly and then you will deserve to be loved, you will be worthy of love, you will be enough." Who wants to run toward con-

ditional love? I mean, this kind of love can wear a woman out. That's not how God loves. God loves unconditionally. He loves me just the way I am. I do not have to do anything for God's love.

I had this limiting belief in my-self, and it was not based on truth. It was based on a little girl's idea of what love was, and it had been limiting me for too long. It was stopping me from being the wife I desired to be because I had so many conditions wrapped up in what love was and was not. For so 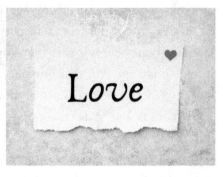 long I felt I was a failure as a mom, that I just couldn't love my children enough—the way they needed to be loved—because of the conditions I put on myself. This ONE limiting belief I uncovered is such an enormous piece of my healing process that I want every woman in the world to know and understand what *unconditional* love is and you, too, can love yourself fully without conditions, expectations, or anything else.

OUR GREATEST NEED

"Love the Lord your God with all your heart and with all your soul and with all your mind and with all your strength.
The second is this: 'Love your neighbor as yourself.'
There is no commandment greater than these."
~ Mark 12:30-31 (NIV)

Our most basic and greatest need is to be loved. We will do just about anything to feel loved. Looking back, I can see how love is the thread woven throughout my life story.

Through this journey, I have realized how often I have pushed love away because of my limiting beliefs created from trauma as a little girl. I know I am not alone—so many little girls, teenagers, and women have been hurt and those *hurts* land our pennies in the mud on the *"tails"* side—the side of fear: Fear of loving others and being hurt. Fear of what love is and what we must do to receive that love. We are living double-minded and the back-and-forth between what we desire and what we are afraid of keeps us in this state of spiritual unrest. Love is the greatest gift we can receive, but we must receive it with open arms and an open heart—no conditions. Love is also the greatest gift we can give with open arms and an open heart—no conditions.

MOVING FORWARD

"It's not the events in our lives that shape us,
rather our beliefs about what those events mean."
~ Tony Robbins

We can let our limiting beliefs formed from the events and experiences in our lives dictate our present and our future, or we can move forward. We have the magnificent gift of free will, which allows us to decide what we are going to believe, no matter what has happened. No matter if you were raped, molested, beaten, cheated on, abandoned, or rejected, you have the choice to see it only from one side or you can choose to Flip the Penny and see the other side for what it is and what you have gained from the experience.

I know this is difficult, but I also know traveling down the "normal" road is hard too. No one can take your faith, your hope, your self-love, or your joy without your permission. You can believe you are worthy, wonderful, strong because God says you are. You can believe no matter what health issue you have had in the past, whether it is fat on your body, physical pain, or disease, from this moment forward, change is possible. When we use the Flip the Penny Principle and flip fear to love, our healing begins. Using affirmations like "I am Self-disciplined" and "I am Loved Unconditionally" are two ways to grow your roots deep, your trunk sturdy, and your fruit a blessing to all.

NEXT STEP

A researcher at Stanford Medical School wrote our heart issues (he identifies them as our beliefs) are the source of almost 100 percent of illness and disease, and if you heal the heart issue, even genetic issues can heal.[5]

Similarly, UT Southwestern University Medical Center in Dallas reported findings healing the issues of the heart (identified as *cellular memories*) is our best hope for healing incurable illness and disease.

"Unconditional love, extended to others without exception, is considered to be one of the highest expressions of spirituality," wrote Montreal University Professor Mario Beauregard, who led a study on the effects of unconditional love on the body. "The rewarding nature of unconditional love facilitates the creation of strong emotional links. Such robust bonds may contribute to the survival of the human species."

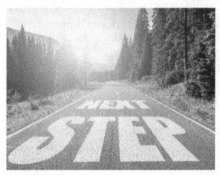

I believe from my experience and the research I found the "S-Spiritual" in the ExSEPshNL Formula is loving God, others, and yourself unconditionally, and the most important next step you can take towards holistic health. *How?* Using the *Flip the Penny Principle* to change Limiting Beliefs to Empowering Beliefs every time you find a roadblock on your journey to bring true healing to your spiritual core, your heart, your beliefs, your relationship with God and to have true harmony in yourself.

**Go to www.shawnacale.com/book-bonus
Printable Journal Pages and Bonus Resources
to Live an Exceptional Life.**

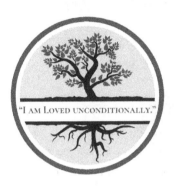

"I AM LOVED UNCONDITIONALLY."

EXERCISE: UNCONDITIONAL LOVE

1. Say the words "I am loved unconditionally." How do you feel about saying those words? Do you feel those words are your truth? If not, this may be an indicator you have the limiting belief—love is conditional. Start with "I choose unconditional love" as a daily affirmation.

Advanced:

1. Using the Flip the Penny Principle find the limiting beliefs that are hiding out in the areas where you're producing unwanted results, acknowledge these are beliefs, not truths, flip them and use them as daily affirmations, pay attention to your thoughts, your words, and when they are not in alignment with the empowering belief continue to repeat the affirmation.

ExSEPshNL Formula: Next Step—Love Yourself Unconditionally.

SPECIAL NOTE:

"You are the light of the world. A town built on a hill cannot be hidden.
Neither do people light a lamp and put it under a bowl.
Instead they put it on its stand, and it gives light to everyone in the house.
In the same way, let your light shine before others,
that they may see your good deeds and glorify your Father in heaven."
~ Matthew 5:14-16 NIV

I believe our only hope is in Jesus Christ, who loves us unconditionally. When we recognize our own limiting beliefs and love ourselves unconditionally the way the Lord loves us, we too can be a light to others. Just a few weeks after I flipped my limiting belief, conditional love, to the empowering belief of unconditional love, a friend commented to me I was glowing. I had seen a picture of myself with my family just days after my experience, and the words "Let your light shine before others" came to my mind. This is when I realized my limiting belief had been snuffing out my light for the world to see for far too long.

If you have accepted the gift of salvation from Jesus Christ and have a relationship with God the Father, the Bible assures us He makes us new. He completely transforms us from the inside out. If you have not accepted the gift of salvation, perhaps today is the day to take this step. Romans 10:9 says all you need to do is *"openly declare that Jesus is the Lord and believe in your heart that God raised him from the dead, you are saved."*

Dear Heavenly Father,

I am grateful for the unconditional love You have given me and all You have done for me in my life. I am ready to accept your gift of salvation. I know I am a sinner and need your forgiveness. I believe in my heart that Jesus Christ died on the cross for my sins and rose from the dead to give me eternal life.

Jesus Christ, please come into my heart and live within me as my Lord and Savior. Direct me on the path You created for me as I live out my days for You.

Amen.

8

The Emotional Connection

"The value of emotions comes from sharing them, not just having them."
~ Simon Sinek

As we continue on our journey with the ExSEPshNL Formula, our next stop is "E" for Emotional health—our emotions, feelings, and relationships with others. The reason I shared my whole story, not just the *"heads"* side, is I wanted to build a foundational—relationship with you. I want you to find emotional freedom as I have. I could have kept my feelings to myself and just shared how to release your own emotional baggage. But that's not what I wanted this book to be about. I feel the emotional connection is missing for so many of us today. I believe if we want true holistic health—freedom, then the emotional connection within ourselves between our spirit and our body must join, and when that happens our connection with God and people will grow even stronger.

> ExSEPshNL Solution: Freedom

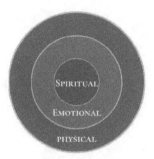

What is an emotional connection?

The picture the Lord gave me was our emotions either connect or disconnect our spiritual being from our physical being. In the SEP Circle, it's the next ring after the center and what joins to our physical being ring. What I find even more interesting is that our spiritual core, our heart—connects to our physical body, our heart—through our emotions. *How?* I like how Candice Pert explains it: *"Emotions are the glue that holds the cells of the organism together."* [1]

Our emotions also connect us with others to build strong bonds. *What if our connections with others exist to teach us how to love? What if we can't love others unconditionally until we first love ourselves unconditionally?* These are thoughts to ponder as we continue to walk and talk about emotional health.

In the Belief Circle, I shared our beliefs lead to our thoughts and our thoughts lead to our emotions. Can a belief also be an emotion and vice versa? I am going to say yes and no. Yes, in the sense that how we love can be a belief as discussed in the previous chapter—conditional and unconditional love. But is love an emotion? Well, this is something I have been contemplating since Junior High School. I remember writing a poem that started: *Love—Is it an emotion or just a notion?* I don't remember the rest of the poem, but this line has been replaying in my mind for over 30 years. A "notion" is another word for *belief*—I doubt I knew that in Junior High, but as you can see, I've been asking questions and seeking answers for many years.

If all emotions stem from love or fear—does that mean love and fear are also emotions or just the roots from which the emotions come? Now I don't share this to confuse you, but to help you see there are many facets to how this whole emotional connection premise works. As we unravel it and understand it better for ourselves, emotional healing and freedom can occur.

E-MOTION

"Emotion is energy in motion."
~ Peter McWilliams

What is an emotion? Well, I learned early in my journey that e-motion is energy in motion.[1] Our thoughts create this energy. We have thousands and thousands of thoughts each day. Our thoughts create emotions by sending out chemicals (neurotransmitters and hormones) that move through our brain—our nervous system using protein tree-like memory structures called dendrites that branch off the cell of the neuron. (I love how the tree analogy just keeps popping up even in the brain.)

As these messages move throughout our nervous system, we have a physical response. Our heart rate increases, our eyes may become dilated, we may flush, we may breathe heavily, we may smile, we may frown, we may become relaxed, or we may cry, laugh, scream or have goosebumps or hives. Positive thoughts and emotions grow our dendrites into beautiful lush trees, while negative thoughts and emotions cause our "memory trees" to become sparse and thorny.[2] While emotions are the physical response, I believe our feelings are the energetic footprint left behind.

What is the purpose of emotions? Emotions tell us something about ourselves and our situation. Created to freely and openly express without judgment, to motivate us, to connect us to God and to others. When we feel an emotion, we can be proactive and respond, or we can be impulsive and reactive based on our emotional intelligence.[3] *Our what?* Yes! That is what I said, the first time I heard those words. I did not understand what the term *emotional intelligence* meant, but then I also did not understand I could control my emotions. *Or did I?* I mean, I went to work and didn't blow up every time things didn't go my way—yet, when I would go home, and my husband or my children said or did something I was like a volcano erupting. Why did I control my emotions sometimes and not others?

Now I shared with you my *White Flour Tortilla Story*, and this is when I realized food played a huge role in the hormonal/emotional roller-coaster I was riding. We have thoughts that produce chemicals; we have hormones that are chemical messengers, and our food is composed of chemicals too. If we get down to it, we have environmental chemicals, often known as *toxins*, that also play a part in this big chemical stew that makes us who we are and affects how we feel.

Just when I thought I understood what I was putting into my body and on my body was affecting my emotions, I had a whole new emotional experience—two emotional releases in one day! My goal in this chapter is to do my best to share with you what I have learned about emotions and the tools I have used to improve my personal emotional intelligence. So, let's start there: *What is emotional intelligence?*

EMOTIONAL INTELLIGENCE

"It is very important to understand that emotional intelligence is not the opposite of intelligence, it is not the triumph of heart over head — it is the unique intersection of both."
~ David Caruso

Emotional intelligence is the ability to relieve stress positively by understanding and managing our emotions. It allows us to use our emotions to build stronger connections, communicate with others, empathize with others, overcome challenges, and even defuse conflict. Emotional intelligence helps us have less stress, feel better, and have more energy. It even helps us succeed in life and achieve our goals. It plays a big part in the last half of our Belief Circle where our emotions lead to our feelings and those feelings lead us into action or even block us from taking action that brings us the results we have.

There are four key areas when looking at emotional intelligence: self-awareness, self-management, social awareness, and relationship management. Each of these is important for our emotional growth and our emotional health. Why do some have higher emotional intelligence than others? Well, that's the question I had, which led me on an emotional journey full of healing.

TRAPPED EMOTIONS

"Trapped emotions are the cause of 90 percent of your problems,
lodging somewhere in your body."
~ Dr. Bradley Nelson

Trapped emotions? Remember from our beliefs come our thoughts and our thoughts create emotions, and these emotions are balls of energy that set off a chemical reaction through our physical body. But when an emotion is not fully felt, is hidden, pushed down, ignored, repressed, or buried, this emotional energy gets trapped. These trapped emotions can and will affect our emotional intelligence.

Different emotions harbor in different areas of the body.[4] When they get trapped in a specific location, they cause havoc to that organ or that area of the body and we find ourselves often in pain, out of balance, or with a disease.

For me, I did not understand I was holding onto trapped emotions. I was an expert at stuffing my emotions and not even aware of what I was doing. When I would hear someone ask, *"Is that emotion serving you?"* It confused me—how could an emotion do anything for me? My entire goal was *not* to feel if I didn't have to. Of course, I wanted to feel all the wonderful emotions—happy, joy, excitement, etc. I would go to my doctor and say, "I just want to *feel* better." I didn't even know what feeling better looked like, I just knew I didn't feel good. But, I didn't understand what I was feeling was the consequences of stuffing my emotions for so long, and not allowing myself to feel both sides of the coin.

I dealt with right lower back pain for almost 20 years, thinking the entire time that the pain was structural and that I just needed to find the physical solution to fix it. With almost 20 years of experience as a physical therapist and helping lots of people with back issues, I just could not understand why I couldn't fix my own pain.

That one day—that one emotional release for the emotion "difficulty" changed my life. Not only did it take away the pain, but it also changed my life in that I could no longer deny my emotions. It was time to feel again. It was time to embrace the emotions when they came, and it was time to capture my thoughts so that the emotions I had could serve me in a way to build up connections and not tear them down.

Now, I am still a work in progress. I still hide emotions and pretend, avoid, and deny the uncomfortable ones; it's a defense mechanism I have had for many years—it's my safe place. But I am getting better, I am allowing myself to feel sad; I am allowing myself to get mad; I accept life can be difficult. Self-awareness is the first step. When I can love myself enough to feel my emotions, listen to them, and learn from them, they can move through and out of my body. I can let go instead of holding on and allowing them to get trapped.

I remember once hearing to heal, you must feel. Emotions need to be expressed to be processed. For so long I held my emotions until I felt I couldn't hold them any longer. It was like a volcano just waiting to erupt. I was so afraid of showing my emotions that I only made it worse by resisting them—this caused the emotional/hormonal roller coaster I was on for far too long.

Feeling your emotions does not mean you have to yell, scream, and become a monster. That is not a healthy way to release. It means when your heart hurts; you look at the situation and what you are thinking and how you feel, and how you can best respond in the situation. It looks like accepting; I am going to be sad and in a state of grief when someone passes away, and to feel the sadness and be okay with the feeling at that moment. Maybe it looks like crying and releasing it through tears. It could look like taking deep breaths and letting it go. Journaling and writing feelings on paper, going for a walk to clear one's head. There are so many ways we can release emotions in a healthy way.

FEELINGS

"Lonely is not being alone, it's the feeling that no one cares."
~ Unknown

An emotion only lasts about 6 seconds from the initial chemical burst to the time it's broken down.[5] Now you may say, *my emotions last way longer than 6 seconds.* What is interesting is our opportunity lies in those 6 seconds, it is what we do with that emotion that leaves the footprint we feel, the actions we take, and the results we receive. Remember me by the trash can yelling at my husband? Something triggered an emotion and because of a deeper trapped emotion I did not want to let go of whatever triggered me, so my thoughts continued regarding that trigger until I created more emotions (physiological responses) more feelings, and more actions—yelling and screaming.

So often we believe we can't *change* how we feel because it's just who we are, or worse, we accept that which we believe someone else thinks we are. Your feelings are yours and yours alone.

We often think it is "normal" to feel the way we do because of a certain situation or because someone has told us to feel a specific way. We often hold on to hate or unforgiveness because of past trauma. It often stems from a belief we formed as a child, and we don't even understand or question what we are feeling. A feeling is not a fact and does not have to be acted upon. No screaming required.

I know feelings can be uncomfortable and overwhelming. In the past, I was the queen of not wanting to feel. But what if our feelings have a function? Though we don't have to obey them, we don't have to ignore them either. Feelings have a purpose, and that purpose may be to help guide you to what you need.

Think of a feeling as an alarm, ask yourself why it's going off? Is it to motivate you to move into action or is it holding you back? Is this a feeling you want to feel tomorrow and the next day, or have you learned what you need to from that feeling today? You get to choose whether you want to change the feeling. *How?* That's the amazing part—we can always go back to the top of the Belief Circle when we are ready to change our feelings.

What if... What if we stopped fighting and judging what we are feeling and accepted and loved that feeling at the moment? What if we listened to that feeling and the story it is telling us? What if we learned from that feeling by asking ourselves questions:

"Why do I feel like no one cares?"

"Nobody calls or comes over."

"Do I call others or go to them?"

"Do I let people care for me?"

"Do I care for others?"

"Do I deserve to be cared for?"

What if we conclude we have been living with the limiting belief "I am not worthy" and that is why we are feeling like *no one cares*?

When we have the belief, "I am not worthy" our thoughts ruminate on this belief. We don't see our worth, our value, and so we stay away from others and find ourselves *alone* because we think they will see our unworthiness. These thoughts bring up the emotion of loneliness and the chemicals pour through our bodies—we fold forward and hide from those near. This leaves us with the feeling that *no one cares*, and the Belief Circle continues.

When we use the *Flip the Penny Principle* and flip "I am not worthy" to "I am worthy" and capture the negative thoughts as soon as they come to the surface—change within will occur.

When reading those words, did you think, but I'm not worthy?

> Affirmation: "I Am Worthy."

Can I just tell you right now—you are worthy! That truth you have been believing has been a lie. Nowhere will you find a book, a report, or a message from the Lord saying you are not worthy. You get to *flip that penny* from the "tails" side and see your full worth. The emotion from this new empowering belief will trickle these amazing chemicals such as oxytocin through your dendrites, growing them to these beautiful trees that make you smile, laugh, and feel like a million bucks. That feeling doesn't have to go away. It can motivate and inspire you to be all that God created you to be. All because you loved and accepted that feeling, you listened and learned to ask yourself questions to find the limiting belief and believed, "I am worthy."

EMOTIONAL BAGGAGE

"Emotional baggage is the elephant in the living room in Western medicine."
~ Dr. Bradley Nelson

I am thinking it will be no surprise to you after reading my story I had some emotional baggage I needed to release. Those trapped emotions that I stored for as long as I can remember were causing my health issues. After I had the emotional release in front of a class full of people, it felt like a load (elephant size) had released from my shoulders, back, and my entire body. I had experienced a similar feeling when I changed my diet and felt like I could handle so much more; putting the two together, I was a new woman.

It was March 2012, and I knew that it was only the beginning of letting go of emotional baggage I had been holding onto way too long. Now believe me when I say I like easy. I like to do something once, mark it off the list and move on to the next project, idea, or dream. But what I realized is this was not a one-and-done type of practice. It's kind of like saying I prayed once, and I'm done. I knew I would spend the rest of my life not only releasing emotions in the present but letting go of the trapped emotions of the past.

There are many techniques to let go of emotional baggage. I, myself, have studied many and I know those are just a few of what is out there. What I don't want you to get caught up in is the right way, the fastest way, the best way, the only way. When I let go of finding THE way, the Lord led me on a journey I am passionate to go down for the rest of my life. I learned to ask questions, and He has put one stone at a time right in front of me, right when I needed it, to release what I was ready to release when I was ready to release it.

I was told once if you don't understand or believe something instead of throwing it out, put it up on a shelf until you are ready. I can't tell you how many things I have put on shelves over the past 10 years, and how many times I have just walked past the book, the memory, or the person I had placed on that shelf only to hear a whisper, *"It's time."* I would then take that technique, tool, or listen to that call or read that book and find the answer to the question I had just asked.

My hope is this book will be a starting point for you to release your own personal emotional baggage. If there are tools that you are not ready to use, it's okay to set it on a shelf. You may find later is the perfect time.

How are you letting go of emotional baggage?

EMOTIONAL RELEASE

"Knowing that if there was a question,
there had to be an answer,
I set out to discover the most effective
ways of healing and maintaining health."
~ Carolyn L. Mein, D.C.

As I've shared before, I love books. Even resource books I read from the front to the back, every page, nothing left unturned. But that doesn't mean I believe everything I read in books. I test what I read to the Word of God, and if I don't understand the author's perspective, that's okay. You may not agree with everything I have written in this book, and I respect that. For me, to read what others think and not shut down because it goes against my beliefs shows me I have grown. Just a few short years ago, I would argue with anyone that did not agree with me or my current beliefs. Now I can listen, learn, and choose what to do with that information and move from there.

One of the resource books I've chosen to use is *Releasing Emotional Patterns with Essential Oils* by Carolyn L. Mein, D.C. I'm not sure if it's because it was the first book I used when releasing my lower back pain, or if it's because I love that she has an emotion, the other side, the way out, the essential oil and the alarm point all in one location.

Early on, I just wasn't sure about all this emotional release stuff. Even after I had experienced it, I had questions. *Is this biblical? Is this of the Lord?* In my search of answers to my questions, I came upon Matthew Chapter 12 verses 43-44 where it talks about the evil spirits leaving and returning to an empty but clean home with seven more evil spirits. I don't know about you, but I don't want to clean my house, only to have it seven times worse. The picture the Lord gave me is an emotion that lives within me does not just need to be released but also needs to be replaced. Just like the penny—there will always be heads and tails, darkness and light, good and evil, and with emotions what many of us call positive and negative. But do I want to just release sadness, or do I want to move to the other side and have joy? This concept of releasing that which no longer serves me—for example, sadness and moving towards joy is also found in the Word.

"For his anger endureth but a moment; in his favour is life: weeping may endure for a night, but joy cometh in the morning."
PSALM 30:5 (KJV)

God does not promise emptiness, He promises the good things in life. I choose to let go and move forward to the promises God has for me. That means I didn't want to just let go of: abandonment, addiction, being alone, anger, and argumentativeness. I wanted to move toward the other side: at-one-ment, freedom, connection, laughter, and peace.

At first, I didn't understand the *way out*—but as I repeated affirmations and learned more about how our core beliefs affect our thoughts and our emotions; I was feeling the shift. One day as I was reading 1 Corinthians 10:13 (NIV) ~ *"No temptation has overtaken you except what is common to mankind. And God is faithful; he will not let you be tempted beyond what you can bear. But when you are tempted, he will also provide a way out so that you can endure it."* I realized God had given me the answers in the Word. He has called me to capture my thoughts, renew my mind (words) and He will always provide a *way out*. Do you remember the exit definition I gave you in Chapter 6? *Exit: A way out, a door, to leave, to depart, an outcome.* I believe we have been given an exit—a *way out* using the Flip the Penny Principle and *flipping* a limiting belief to an empowering belief, and I use affirmations, scriptures, and worship music to do it.

Then there are essential oils. I spent almost a year using essential oils for myself and my family's physical bodies before ever learning I could use them with releasing emotional patterns. The results we had were amazing. No longer did I feel I needed to use toxic products or over-the-counter drugs to keep my family healthy. I could use something all-natural that came from the plants God created for me and you. But when I went to the CARE Intensive, I also learned how these oils affected our limbic system (our emotional center) and helped our physical body make changes. Remember, emotions are energy (natural chemicals made in our bodies and created from our thoughts) and essential oils also have a frequency and are a natural chemical made in plants. *How do we change energy?* What if we used another energy source? Think about how we flip a penny. Will that penny just flip over by itself? No, we must use energy—our hand—to flip it over. I have found using affirmations, scriptures, and positive words work, but adding essential oils and deep breathing amplifies it. Let me get sciencey with you for just a moment. When essential oil molecules travel through our nasal passage to a neuron receptor, it is then transported straight to the limbic brain, the hypothalamus which plays a part in the release of hormones and not only is it more enjoyable than drugs, it has become a daily practice for many with life-changing results.

Third, but not least, is when I researched more about emotions being stored in our body—the heart, the lungs, the lower back, the liver. It was so interesting to see how the emotion *alone* is stored in the heart, *fear* in the lungs, *not being supported* in the lower back, and *anger* in the liver. The research took me to stories of those who had cancer and had so much *hate* stored within and refused to forgive and died of their cancer. Then there were those who forgave and found healing through the process. Using essential oils at the alarm point helps me to remember why I don't want to push my emotions down, why I want to feel them fully, and what trapped emotions actually do to my physical body all the way down to the cellular level. When I anoint myself with oils, I am allowing the energy from the essential oils to work in the location the emotion has been trapped at an energetic level. This process has opened my eyes to the connection between my spiritual, emotional, and physical being and how they are all one to make me who I am and you who you are.

I often have people ask me, "How do you know emotional release works?" "How long does it take?" My answer is always, "All I know is that it has worked for me." It worked for me that very first time when I didn't even believe it could. Even though I was resistant—taking the action allowed me to have the most amazing result—I have now been pain-free in my right lower back since 2012, and I had dealt with that pain for almost 20 years.

I also know I spent 30 or more days, multiple times, over a 3-year period releasing anger, and did not know if it was working. Then one day when my family was traveling, we went to a pizza place, and my youngest son, Bryce, spilled his water. I kind of laughed and handed him a napkin and said, "You might want to clean that up before you get wet." My oldest son, Ryan, just looked at me and said, "Are you not going to get mad and yell at him?" I answered back, "It's okay; he just spilled water." But it was at that moment I realized in the past something as minor as spilled water would have been an emotional trigger and sent me in a tailspin. I would have gotten angry and everyone in the pizza place would have known it, felt it, and heard it too.

The funny thing is, the other side of anger is laughter and that is what I had done—laughed. The thought not only had I removed the anger, but I had laughter in its place, allowed me to see I was healing. It may not have been as quick as the first time, nor as powerful of an emotional release as the second time. But, Wow! How many other emotions had I released and not even been aware of, because it was now just a part of the new me—the exceptional me?

"What emotions would you like to release?"

EMOTIONAL TRIGGERS

"Avoiding your triggers isn't healing.
Healing happens when you are triggered and you're able
to move through the pain, the pattern, and the story—
and walk your way to a different ending."
~ Vienna Pharaon

I imagine trapped emotions looking like a red fiery ball swirling and swirling, waiting to move into action. Then something triggers the emotion, a person, a place, a smell, and it's like the energetic ball ignites and goes bouncing and hitting everything in its way and causes even more energetic damage and pain than the first time.

Before I learned about emotional release, I would try to control my life in a way that prevented me from being triggered. Sometimes it meant spending time alone and away from those I loved most to protect myself and them from my emotional outbursts. Other times I would try to control the people around me so they didn't trigger me. It wasn't the people or the circumstances or the situations—I learned it was me. Trauma I had not dealt with; emotions I had been hiding because I thought it was safer than dealing with them.

One thing I learned by writing my Penny Story is that a lot of the things I did and didn't do were to feel safe. In Psychology 101—Maslow's Hierarchy of Needs the lowest rung on the pyramid is Physiological Needs—food, water, a roof overhead, clothing, and I have always had those things.

MASLOW'S HIERARCHY OF NEEDS

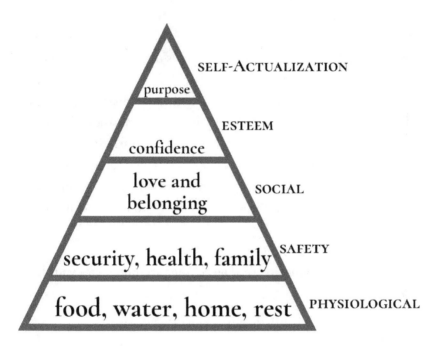

The next rung is Safety Needs—As I walked through my story, I saw times in my childhood when my beliefs were being formed; life was unstable, unknown, and unsafe. We can often get stuck on a rung and cannot work our way up to the next one until we have dealt with the trapped emotions.

The third rung is Social and includes love and belonging, the fourth is Esteem, and the very top is what Maslow calls *Self-Actualization,* or we might call *Self-Awareness.* Often, we must start at the bottom rung, and flip limiting beliefs and/or release emotions blocking us from moving up the hierarchy allowing us to reach the top.

I had the honor of attending one of Carolyn L. Mein's workshops, and she gave us this beautiful visual of walking across a bridge to the other side when releasing emotions.

I remember a time when I blew up with my daughter Emily and later questioning what it was I was feeling. Wanting to blame Emily, but knowing it wasn't her but a trapped emotion she had triggered. I grabbed my book *Releasing Emotional Patterns with Essential Oils* and looked up the emotion: *frustration.* I then took my lemon essential oil and breathed it in deep as I imagined a bridge—it was one of those big red covered bridges and I could see Jesus on the other side. He was who I was walking towards as I was letting go of *frustration* and saying the affirmation in the book. It felt so good to not blame my daughter for making me feel a certain way because the truth is nobody has that much control over me. Only I have control over myself. It also felt good not to beat myself up for getting upset. The trigger became my teacher and showed me an area I still needed to work on. I keep an Emotional Health Worksheet to track the emotions I need to release—this has become a daily practice.

What are some emotional triggers you have noticed in your life?

TRAUMA

"ACEs are a game changer.
Unless you fix the trauma... the hole in the soul...
where the wounds started, you're working at the wrong thing...
[The ACE story is] HUGE... and I've done a lot of stories in my time."
~ Oprah Winfrey

On my journey, I came across ACEs—Adverse Childhood Experiences Study[6] that has researched over half a million people since 1998. The ACE study examines 10 types of trauma between birth and 18 years of age and found the higher the ACE score, the higher risk for emotional and physical health conditions, and for the leading causes of death in the United States. When I took the ACE test myself, I scored high enough that it showed I was at high risk for chronic disease.

Many women just want to better understand why they feel the way they feel emotionally and physically. Why they may be sick, why they're not getting better, why stress seems to trigger symptoms, and why medications rarely work or even make symptoms worse.

The study found an ACE score of 4 or more increased the likelihood of chronic pulmonary lung disease by 390 percent; hepatitis, 240 percent; depression, 460 percent, and attempted suicide by 1,220 percent.

They found people with higher ACE scores were hungry for self-awareness, craved connection, and wanted to be seen, valued, and understood. They wanted to know they mattered. They found those with higher scores disconnect from themselves and from others. I can agree personally with all those findings.

What they found is when children are overloaded with stress hormones, they're in a *fight, flight,* or *freeze* mode, which makes long-lasting changes to their brains and their nervous systems. This increases their chances of chronic diseases such as obesity, diabetes, asthma, autoimmune diseases, sleep disorders, and many more. But there is hope. Knowing about ACEs has helped doctors and patients better understand how chronic issues stem from stress. Instead of using drugs, they can empower themselves with stress-reducing techniques that can turn lives around and bring in more joy and holistic health.

Knowing this information has helped me in multiple ways. I realized if *stress* from trauma has been my *normal,* then I may not be aware that I am stressed and must not wait until I *feel* stressed to use the tools and techniques available to lower my stress levels. It has also helped me see how important it is for me to release emotions that have been expending my energy and affecting my health.

> Trauma is stored as stress in the body.

Go to www.shawnacale.com/book-bonus
Printable Journal Pages and Bonus Resources
to Live an Exceptional Life.

ACTION: ACE TEST

1. If you have had trauma in your life, take the ACE test online.[7]

2. Did your ACE score surprise you? How are you going to use this information to help you?

STRESS

"The greatest weapon against stress
is our ability to choose one thought over another."
~ William James

What is stress? Everyone talks about it, but do we understand what it is and where it comes from? First, let's recognize that there are several types of stress. There is spiritual stress, emotional stress, and physical stress. Spiritual stress occurs when we are out of harmony and our beliefs are not in agreement with one another. We have already learned our spiritual being is connected to our emotional being and the two can and will affect one another. This means spiritual stress may cause emotional stress. The same with our emotional being connected to our physical being, we will see emotional stress affecting our physical being. Let's dive into emotional stress in this chapter and we will discuss physical stress in the next chapter.

Emotional stress is an emotion—energy in motion—with a physiological response affecting heart rate and hormones in a way that stresses the body. We often think of the stress hormone, *cortisol*, rising as one of these signs. Research has linked ninety percent or more of diseases to the body's inability to handle stressors.

Everyone has a different threshold on how much they can handle before they become stressed. I have shared when I was in my late 30s I woke up feeling "done" before I even got started. Things a few years before that would not have bothered me set me off big time. When we hold on to trapped emotions and trauma, it takes up space, it uses up our energy. We try to add in the good things of life, but often it feels there is just no room. I pictured if I were a tree, my tree trunk was skinny, and my roots were very shallow, and anything coming my way seemed like a storm that would break me. The true storm was within me.

I have shared ways we can grow deeper roots: walking, prayer, gratitude, flipping limited beliefs, increasing our emotional intelligence by releasing trapped emotions... and I will share more. What I want you to understand right now: when we are living in a high stressed state we are becoming weaker spiritually, emotionally, and physically. Stressors can strengthen us, being stressed creates disease.

What can you do to let go of stress? My pastor, Craig Groeschel, says: "*Life will always move in the direction of our strongest thoughts.*" [8] So, when you are feeling stressed and anxious, it's time to consider what questions you're asking yourself, what thoughts you're focusing on, and what limiting beliefs may bring on these thoughts? This is my favorite scripture to meditate on when anxious or stressed out.

> "*Do not be anxious about anything, but in every situation, by prayer and petition, with thanksgiving, present your requests to God. And the peace of God, which transcends all understanding, will guard your hearts and your minds in Christ Jesus.*"
>
> PHILIPPIANS 4:6-7 (NIV)

Another tool I have found helpful when I am stressed is to use a technique I learned at a physical therapy continuing education course: EFT—Emotional Freedom Technique, also known as *tapping*.[9] When we are stressed, our energy is out of balance. Using acupuncture points and tapping these points disturbs the current energy (emotion) and may help decrease stress and restore balance. A study published in the *Journal of Nervous and Mental Disease*, the oldest peer-reviewed psychology journal in the United States, EFT lowered the major stress hormone cortisol significantly more than other interventions tested.[10] The goal with EFT is to rate your stress level and to tap until the number decreases to a level you feel more comfortable with. I have found this to be a great tool when I am *feeling* stressed about something specific in my life.

Go to www.shawnacale.com/book-bonus
Printable Journal Pages and Bonus Resources
to Live an Exceptional Life.

ACTION: EFT

1. If you find your stress levels are high and you are aware of your stress, learn more about EFT.[11]

2. Follow an EFT Tapping Session Video and journal about your results.[12]

FIGHT, FLIGHT, AND FREEZE

"The amygdala in the emotional center sees and hears everything
that occurs to us instantaneously and is the trigger point
for the fight or flight response."
~ Daniel Goleman

I have known about stress and the *fight, flight,* and *freeze* response for years. It is something I studied and discussed with my patients, but I did not understand what I was feeling and going through was just that—stress. I was so out of touch and disconnected from my emotions; I didn't even know I was having anxiety attacks until several years into my healing process. At the time I would just say, "I feel like an elephant is on my chest." I could feel the physical aspect but couldn't define the emotional. I just knew there was something wrong, and I didn't feel good and I wanted to feel better.

The stress response begins in the brain and our senses send the information to our amygdala, an area in the brain that processes our emotions. When it perceives danger, it sends a distress signal to the hypothalamus—the emotional command center—and it releases the chemicals and hormones for the *fight* and *flight* responses through the sympathetic nervous system (one branch of the autonomic nervous system).

Our sympathetic nervous system signals our adrenal glands that provide us the burst of energy to respond to danger—similar to pushing the gas pedal in a car. This happens so fast you are not even aware of what is going on. If nothing is done to reset the autonomic system and activate the parasympathetic system (the flip side), there is nothing putting on the brakes and allowing rest to occur. You are then stuck in a chronic stress cycle. With time this becomes your "normal" and like most cars, at some point, you will run out of gas.

I remember spending my days fighting with my husband, my kids, and anyone else that wanted to argue with me. I was in this constant *fight* stage and was not even aware. I didn't like how I felt, and I would feel bad for fighting with everyone, but it's what I did *automatically*, and I felt like it was the entire world against me.

The adrenaline hormones being released got me out of bed and got things done, but it wasn't fun and it sure wasn't pretty. I felt as if I could just stay and *fight* it out; maybe at some point, I would win and everything would be okay. But I was tired, worn out, and when there was no clear winner I got to a point where I didn't want to fight anymore. Though this is a natural response meant to be used when we need to fight to save our life. My response was *not* natural, it turned my sympathetic nervous system *on* and I desperately needed to turn it *off*. I wish someone had explained to me that what I was feeling, and what was going on inside was the stress response. But all I knew to do was go to my doctor, who wanted to put me on antidepressants. I didn't feel depressed and just ended up fighting him on taking a drug to fix a problem he called "normal."

Antidepressants are synthetic chemicals that work to make chemical changes in the body. For many, this is the only solution they know, because it's the only solution given to them. The problem is they don't fix the root cause and often there are as many side-effects as issues they help. Early on my journey when I was researching how food affects emotions, I found Kelly Brogan, MD, a holistic psychiatrist who had a free e-book called *Change Your Food, Heal Your Mood—3 Steps to a Happier Body and a Healthier Brain.*[13] I found so much information in this little e-book that really helped me better understand how much food really affected how I felt. She is also the author of the *New York Times* bestseller—*A Mind of Your Own: The Truth About Depression and How Women Can Heal Their Bodies to Reclaim Their Lives.*[14] Both books have been instrumental resources in my healing process.

In my story, I share how one day I was just done fighting and all I could think about was running, running far, far, away. I felt like a terrible wife, mother, daughter, and friend. How could I tell anyone how I was feeling? Again, I never thought, *Could this feeling be stress?* I was now in the *flight* stage and my body was responding to danger to run, but the only danger was self-inflicted. There was no bear or tiger or anything else chasing me, so I stayed put and my energy continued to wane, and I felt less and less like myself and more and more like a stranger.

Then after my third miscarriage I was told that it would take time to get my strength, my energy and it was all "normal," but by then I had nothing to give, I was no longer in the sympathetic *fight* and *flight* stage, I have since learned I had moved to the parasympathetic *freeze* stage. I felt numb, and I was so dissociated from myself and those around me. Though I was not taking any drugs, my body was producing its own analgesic chemicals to protect me from the danger my body thought it was in. Think of how a possum pretends to be dead as a self-defense mechanism. This was me.

Chronic stress causes major issues. It does not allow us to balance. Again, let me reiterate: Most women don't even know they are in a chronic stress state. That was me. And maybe you. We all move in and out of the acute stress state, but our body can only handle so much and at some point, we begin to feel stress is the "norm" and it sticks right there and becomes the chronic stress state. There is no more nervous system reset, bringing you back to a balanced state.

Stress causes the brain to shrink, energy production in the mitochondria (energy powerhouse) slows down, and the cells of the body go into protection mode as self-defense. Healing can only occur when the cells are making energy. **I was depleted.**

I often hear women say, "I'm not that stressed." Yet, they have a list of chronic diseases such as obesity, high blood pressure, high blood-sugar levels, high heart rate... all telltale signs of a chronic stress state. They give us medication to stop, block, and prevent the symptoms, but as long as we are in the chronic stress state, our body cannot heal.

Are you in a chronically stressed state?
Do you relate more to the *fight, flight,* or *freeze* state?

VAGAL RESPONSE

"Stimulating the vagus nerve sends acetylcholine, throughout the body,
not only relaxing you, but also turning down the fires of inflammation."
~ Dr. Mark Hyman

Stressed out has become the "norm". Over 55 percent of Americans are stressed during the day.[15] What do we do to get unstressed? That was the question I had when I heard about the vagal response. Then I researched the Polyvagal Theory by Dr. Stephen Porges[16], and it helped me to better understand the entire stress response I shared earlier. I hope this will help you understand it too and, better yet, what you can do to help yourself get out of the stressed state.

We have what we call a *vagus nerve*, which is the longest and most complex cranial nerve in our body, and it comprises thousands of sensory fibers that make up our sense called *neuroception*—this specific sense decides whether something is safe or dangerous. The vagus nerve connects our brain to the rest of the body and is often known as the "heart-brain connection."

Our vagus nerve works as a brake during an acute stressed state. When we are in *fight* or *flight* and the gas is on full throttle, the vagus nerve, when it feels safe, brings balance to the body. But when our body gets into a chronically stressed state, it becomes more difficult to reset and turn on the brakes.

Did you catch the words "feels safe?" When we are stuck on Maslow's Hierarchy rung of Safety Needs, it's not about *if* we are safe, it's about what our body feels *is* safe.

Just like there are two sides to a coin, we have two sides of our vagus nerve. If we *fight* hard enough or run far enough that our body feels safe, the ventral side of the vagus nerve will move into the healing state. If the dorsal side feels we are in extreme danger, we will shut down and move into the *freeze* state.

The vagus nerve is also responsible for regulating our vital organs such as our heart and plays a part in slowing down the heart rate, lowering blood pressure, lowering inflammation, decreasing depression, and decreasing pain.

We are wired to feel safe when we are loved. If we feel that we have to do something to feel safe and/or loved or have certain expectations to meet (conditional love) then we can find ourselves in a stressed state.

Feeling not loved, abandoned, or any of the other emotions from the fear side will lead us straight to the stressed state. Again, we often see this in women who have high ACE scores.

What can we do to help the vagus nerve? We can increase *vagal tone*, kind of like how we can tone our muscles by using specific exercises. Research has shown prayer to stimulate the vagus nerve. Yoga, deep-breathing techniques, meditation, cold exposure, probiotics, omega-3 fatty acids, massage, walking, laughing and even essential oils help improve vagal tone too.

How do you know if you have a good vagal tone? It's called *heart rate variability*. The higher your vagal tone, the more heart rate variability you have, and the healthier and more resilient your heart is. I remember several years ago getting to play with a biofeedback device through the company HeartMath. I could visually see how my breathing, changing my thoughts, and walking affected my heart rate variability. The breathing and walking didn't surprise me much; you expect it to change your heart rate with activity, but looking at pictures that changed my thoughts—heart variability surprised me and helped me better understand how important our thoughts are to our spiritual core—the heart.

What I have learned in my studies is that the vagus nerve is our emotional connection between our spiritual and physical body—some call it the Silver Cord, I call it the key to the healing state.

 Go to www.shawnacale.com/book-bonus
Printable Journal Pages and Bonus Resources
to Live an Exceptional Life.

ACTION: VAGAL TONE

1. Curious what your vagal tone is? You can find free apps for your smart-phone to give you a stress index score or your heart rate variability.

HEART WALL

"The first step toward healing from anxiety and depression
is to remove the Heart-Wall."
~ Dr. Bradley Nelson

When we walked through the Spiritual Core Chapter, I shared I dove deep on the subject of love after I realized I had a limiting belief—conditional love. But there is more to the story, and unlocking strongholds I had for a long time was a big part of the healing process. When all this happened, I had studied the *Emotion Code* by Dr. Bradley Nelson.[17] I had heard about the book and technique from several people, but my friend Mica was using it and telling me all about her wonderful results. She asked me if I knew about the heart-wall. I asked her to tell me more, and she explained it as trapped emotions (energy) building a wall around the heart to protect it. I told her it sounded like what God had been sharing with me in response to *strongholds* in 2 Corinthians Chapter 10—a limiting belief surrounding my heart was a way to protect my heart. Yet, the Lord was also letting me know I could trust Him to be my stronghold, my protector—it was time to let go of emotional strongholds surrounding my heart and completely trust Him.

I read the book and added it to my emotional toolbox. As I was reading, I knew once again it was God leading me to another answer pertaining to my many questions. A heart-wall makes it difficult to give and receive love, or even feel positive emotions such as joy and happiness, but the negative emotions... it was like a gigantic magnet over my heart that continued to attract layer after layer.

One thing I learned from the book was how to use the *Sway test* to ask first if I had a heart-wall, then how deep, and what substance it was made of. This process helped me to learn that yes, I had a heart-wall, and not just any heart-wall but a 5-mile deep heart-wall made of a metal stronger than steel and had over 1000 trapped emotions. Talk about a tight fortress I had built around my heart to protect me. The question: Who or what did I need to protect myself from? From the questions, I asked: I concluded I built the wall when I was 4 years old and the first emotion to start my heart-wall was *worry*.

I released one heart-wall after another: *helplessness, defensiveness,* and *grief* were just a few. I was pretty surprised by the emotion of *helplessness* until I prayed, and the Lord helped me connect the dots with my story of when I was 10 years old and decided I would never be a victim. Instead, I took the emotion of *helplessness* and stuffed it and took the memory and the blame with me. I let *shame* be the only emotion and feeling I lived by instead of loving and listening to the little girl inside who felt *helpless*. The more I moved forward, the more interesting it got—I released emotions such as *wishy-washy* (sounds like double-minded to me) and *guilt*—I was ecstatic to see those long-time trapped emotions go. I spent a month releasing trapped emotions day after day and made a little progress knocking away layers from my heart wall; I removed at least 100 feet out of my 5-mile fortress. Knowing this would be a lifelong journey, I accepted the fact I would need patience through the healing process.

Until... the week I realized I had the limiting belief of conditional love.

As I released more trapped emotions around my heart, I came to the emotion of *hopelessness*. I asked more questions and got more answers—it was from when I was 12 years old and my parents were getting a divorce. Now the amazing part is when I released this emotion, I felt it. I felt the weight on my shoulders (where I carry my stress) release and I felt tingly all over. My heart-wall had decreased to 485-feet-deep and was now wood.

Now you may read this and think this is crazy or wild or whatever other thought you have formed in your head, but here it is—me sharing with you my story and the journey to healing I have walked through to get where I am today.

I shared with you in my story I had my appendix removed when I was 12 and promised to tell you more. In the *Releasing Emotional Patterns with Essential Oils* book, the emotion connected to the alarm point—appendix—is *disillusioned* and the other side is *substance*.

Disillusioned: "disappointed in someone or something that one discovers to be less good than one had believed."[18]

If you have ever gone through a divorce or a child of divorced parents, I am sure you too have built some limiting beliefs about love. I believe that I became disillusioned regarding love.

I have shared one of my favorite passages in the Bible is 1 Corinthians 13:4-7 (NLT). "*Love is patient and kind...* and ends with *Love never gives up, never loses faith, is always hopeful, and endures through every circumstance.*"

Did you get that? Love is always hopeful! Now you might see where *wishy-washy* may have come from. I had this empowering belief pertaining to God and this wonderful passage on love, yet I had this limiting belief that love may not be all I thought it was. It didn't appear love endured through every circumstance, at least not for my family.

> *"Now faith is the substance of things hoped for, the evidence of things not seen."*
> HEBREWS 11:1 (KJV)

We define *faith* as "a powerful belief in something unseen." For years I did not understand what the word *substance* meant in this verse. Then in 2017, when I was teaching a 30-Day Emotional Health Journey class I remembered Dr. Caroline Leaf, my favorite Cognitive Neuroscientist, says the *substance* is a chemical. She found those who have faith make a different chemical substance in their brain compared to those who do not.[19]

That chemical substance changes our brain. When we have a *hopeful* thought, we change our emotions, which changes our feelings and changes our brain and our life. If you have LOST faith, the substance "HOPE" is where you can start.

> *"We have this hope as an anchor for the soul, firm and secure."*
> HEBREWS 6:19 (NIV)

Our soul is our conscious and subconscious mind—our soul is where our thoughts, emotions, and feelings come from. Hope keeps you steady. Hope keeps you grounded. Hope works with direction and support for you to set and reach inspired goals. Hope can be your anchor when going through a terrible storm. Whether the storm is inside or outside of you, there is hope.

Affirmation: "I Am Hopeful."

Remember when I said I released *hopelessness*. The other side is *hopeful*. I now know when I am *hopeful* I create a chemical that relieves stress and is healing to my body. For me, that was a 4-mile-deep discovery. In the *Releasing Emotional Patterns with Essential Oils* book, the affirmation is, *"There is a way out."* I just shared with you one verse God gives us in the Word about a way out, but did you know there are at least 55 more? Sounds like a lot of HOPE to me. They often list the location for this trapped emotion as bone marrow, spleen, or stomach. When I was going through this process, I remembered I had just been meditating on a scripture a few days before.

> *"For the word of God is quick, and powerful, and sharper than any two-edged sword, piercing even to the dividing asunder of soul and spirit, and of the joints and marrow, and is a discerner of the thoughts and intents of the heart."*
>
> HEBREWS 4:12 (KJV)

What does this scripture even mean? I believe it is saying our soul, which is our thoughts, emotions, and feelings—our spirit, which is the deepest part of us where God dwells, our beliefs/our faith—and our joints and marrow, physical body are all connected. Simply: The Word of God is what allows us to discern our thoughts and get to our hearts and break free from the strongholds (heart walls) stopping us from living an exceptional life.

HEART

*"You can close your eyes to the things you don't want to see,
but you can't close your heart to the things you don't want to feel."*
~ Johnny Depp

I hope you are seeing and feeling the foundation I have been building here within this chapter on Emotional Connection. The heart is the connector. When we build walls (trapped emotions and trauma) around our heart, it affects our spirit and our body. When we go through life, trying not to feel—choosing what we think is bad or good we stop our spiritual heart from growing and we stress out our physical heart.

The ancients believed that the heart was the central organ, and it moved the rest of the body. I agree. Our spiritual heart is where our beliefs begin, these beliefs are where our thoughts originate and those thoughts are so powerful that they create emotion (energy in motion). Each emotion can come and go in a mere 6 seconds. When we listen to the emotion—is it a warning, an alarm, or is it bringing peace and joy? Once we acknowledge what the emotion is, we can choose what we want to do with it. If I choose to hold on to an emotion that is not serving me in a positive way, I will feel the stress the energy causes both emotionally and physically. If I choose to see both sides and move towards the direction that will serve me in a positive way, then I have learned from this emotion and increasing my emotional intelligence.

How we feel day-to-day is based on the emotional footprints left behind. Those feelings motivate and inspire us to the actions that lead us to the results we desire or those feelings put out roadblocks, stopping us from taking action towards our goals and our dreams.

When we can spend more time in a state of peace, our body heals. When we spend more time in a stressed state, our body becomes diseased. Throughout the Bible, there are over 800 scriptures on the heart, and each time I read one I learn how the heart connects all three: our spiritual, emotional, and physical being.

"A merry heart doth good (like) a medicine, but a broken spirit dries up the bones."

PROVERBS 17:22 (KJV)

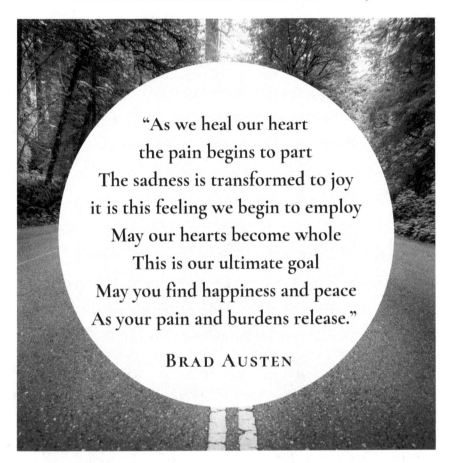

"As we heal our heart
the pain begins to part
The sadness is transformed to joy
it is this feeling we begin to employ
May our hearts become whole
This is our ultimate goal
May you find happiness and peace
As your pain and burdens release."

BRAD AUSTEN

LOVE AND FEAR

"There is no fear in love, but perfect love casts out fear."
~ 1 John 4:18a (ESV)

I asked at the beginning of the chapter if love and fear were emotions. I am not sure what conclusion you may have made at this point regarding this question, but the answer I have found on my journey is that emotions come from our thoughts based on empowering beliefs rooted in love—such as happiness, contentment, peace, and joy; or limiting beliefs rooted in fear—anger, hate, anxiety, and guilt.

We are humans living the human experience on earth. I believe that both love and fear are part of that human experience. Some say darkness is the absence of light; does that mean fear is the absence of love?

God is perfect love. When we find our thoughts, our emotions, our feelings rooted in fear—it leads us down a dark road, we must exit off that road and take the road that leads to love.

> *"For God hath not given us the spirit of fear; but of power, and of love, and of a sound mind."*
>
> 2 TIMOTHY 1:7 (KJV)

I believe fear is our greatest enemy in this world. Our emotions are the road signs showing us the road we are on. When we are spending more time rooted in fear than love, we are traveling the "normal" road that leads us to disease. Many people do not know how to deal with fear and the emotions that arise, so they turn to food, medication, alcohol, and illegal and legal drugs to feel better. But the key to feeling better is choosing love over fear. Every time we use the *Flip the Penny Principle* and choose love over fear, we use the power given to us.

I don't know your "tails" side of the story. What I know is no matter your story, you are worthy of love. Love from another human being is wonderful, but the unconditional love of God is exceptional. God will never give up on you or stop loving you. When you hold the belief—you are unworthy—your heart hardens, and it hides your light. You may think as I thought: *Jesus lives in my heart, isn't that enough? Shouldn't I feel Him, shouldn't my light shine automatically?* But so many of us are holding onto those trapped emotions rooted from fear, and we build a wall and block out that beautiful light from our hearts. We often hold on to them so tight and bury them so deep we don't even realize the hold they have on us.

I shared the story of my pastor telling me my pre-marriage counseling test showed I was *hostile.* For years I had this brain block on that specific word. I could explain it—say it started with an "h"—but could not remember the name. It was like that specific emotion was hidden and I didn't want to deal with it. Recently I had the same thing happen where I could not think of the word *discernment*. I was working on letting go of judgment and I was going to use the affirmation, "I am discerning," every time I judged myself or someone else. It was a grand plan, except every time I would get as far as "I am" and think, "What is that word?" I would say, "I am not judgmental," but I knew that had me focusing on being judgmental. We become what we focus on. I could remember it started with a "d", but I would give up and go find where I wrote the affirmation. After several weeks I could say, "I am discerning" without looking it up. I am telling you the power of words can make some amazing transformations. When the word became easier to pull up to the surface, the more I realized I had become discerning.

So often we need help to find those hidden emotions. We may uncover them when writing our story—that is how I found many. You may need a coach or counselor to walk you through the process—that is how I found others. You may need to have a session with someone who specializes in emotional release, balancing the body and relieving stressors. I want to remind you—you are not alone. Each of us has emotions rooted in fear and love. That does not make you a bad person or wrong or anything else—it makes you human. But as a human you can ask yourself, *Is this emotion driving me, or am I choosing the direction I want to go?*

I had to accept that fear fueled my stress, anxiety, and not love. I had to accept that going to "food"—my drug of choice—was not the answer. I had to listen to the thoughts so I could find where they were coming from. I had to read the road signs and listen to the alarms going off, so I was aware of the road I was traveling, but most of all I had to discern where what I was feeling was rooted—fear or love.

I believe that each of our experiences here on earth is another opportunity to take a step in faith and to learn how to choose love over fear. Love is a choice—the emotions we experience: patience, kindness, forgiveness, gratitude, joy, all come from love. Love leads to emotional connection.

"Let love and faithfulness never leave you; bind them around your neck, write them on the tablet of your heart."

PROVERBS 3:3 (NIV)

Are you ready to have less emotional stress and more energy?

NEXT STEP

According to a study by *The Journal of Health Psychology*, being a forgiving person can reduce your stress levels and boost your mental and physical health. It can improve sleep, lower cholesterol, reduce pain, anxiety, and blood pressure.[20]

It might surprise you, the number of studies on forgiveness. I shared in Chapter 7 the unconditional love God has for each one of us and the gift of forgiveness we can accept at any time. Often, we think about God forgiving us, forgiving others, or others forgiving us, but what studies have found is most people have more difficulty forgiving themselves. Do you want a scientific, proven way to improve your health? *Forgiveness.*

I always thought the opposite of love was hate, but as I shared earlier, the opposite of love is fear and the opposite of hate is forgiveness—rooted in love.

Can I give you a piece of advice? Forgive yourself and others. I know this is difficult. It is something I am still working on each day. All those emotions I shared in my story. How I felt about myself and the feelings I wanted to hide. I hated that little girl inside. I hated what she allowed to happen. Self-hatred brings suffering. I was tired of suffering. I decided it was time to forgive myself, to forgive the little girl inside, who never deserved the trauma she went through, but even more so did not deserve a lifetime of hatred from the woman she had become.

Are you tired of suffering and asking why?
Why am I stressed, hostile, angry?

These are questions, I asked myself for years and the answers I found on my journey lead me to the emotion: *unforgiveness.* This one emotion is linked to high levels of stress and hostility. Neuroimaging shows unforgiveness correlates with anger. Studies even show unforgiveness increases the hormone cortisol and lowers the immune system. However, forgiving oneself increases T-helper cells improving the immune system. Replacing hate with forgiveness may bring you more holistic healing than you ever knew was possible.

How do we forgive ourselves?

Psalm 130:7 in the Passion Translation says, *"O Israel, keep hoping, keep trusting, and keep waiting on the Lord, for he is tenderhearted, kind, and forgiving. He has a thousand ways to set you free!"* If like me you have felt you have done all the things and are still searching for emotional freedom, there is hope. Trust what you have done has been part of the healing process. Each day you have the choice to forgive. Each day you can use a tool, technique, affirmation to remove one more layer that has been blocking you from living the life you were created to live. I have used all the tools I have discussed, and I have found each exercise has helped me become more like Jesus and less like the unforgiving woman of the world. There are many ways to walk this path—all you need to do is take the next step to emotional freedom.

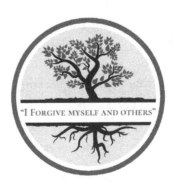

Go to www.shawnacale.com/book-bonus
Printable Journal Pages and Bonus Resources
to Live an Exceptional Life.

EXERCISE: FORGIVENESS

1. **Flip the Penny Principle™:** Remember, all emotions start with our beliefs, and hate is from fear. So, flipping the penny from *fear* to *faith* is a great place to start.

2. **Releasing Emotions:** *Releasing Emotional Patterns with Essential Oils* is a great tool for releasing and replacing an emotion such as hate and moving to the other side—forgiveness.

3. **Emotion Code:** Great tool to uncover any unforgiveness and any other trapped emotions preventing you from forgiving.

4. **AFT—Aroma Freedom Technique:** 12-step process with 7 essential oils with a Certified AFT Practitioner to release unforgiveness.

5. **EFT—Emotional Freedom Technique:** I walked through this process regarding unforgiveness at a physical therapy continuing education course when learning that chronic pain has been found to be related to unforgiveness and without forgiveness, many patients never find the pain relief or healing they are searching for—not through therapy, drugs, or surgery.

6. **Touch for Health:** A balancing session with a goal set to forgive oneself or someone. Locating any stressors blocking this goal from being met using muscle-testing and acupressure touch to correct any imbalances or restrictions.

ExSEPshNL Formula: Next Step—Forgiveness.

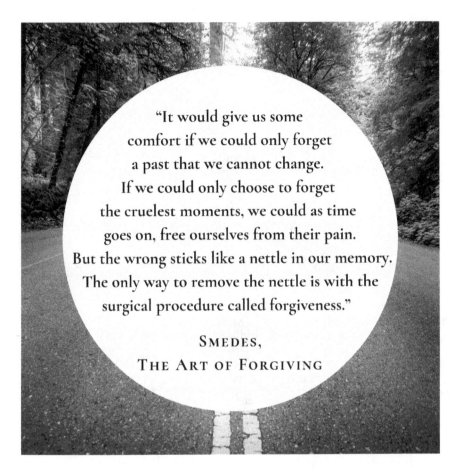

"It would give us some
comfort if we could only forget
a past that we cannot change.
If we could only choose to forget
the cruelest moments, we could as time
goes on, free ourselves from their pain.
But the wrong sticks like a nettle in our memory.
The only way to remove the nettle is with the
surgical procedure called forgiveness."

SMEDES,
THE ART OF FORGIVING

9

The Physical Body

"Take care of your body, it's the only place you have to live."
~Jim Rohn

As we continue with our walk and talk, the next stop in the ExSEPshNL
Formula is the "P" for physical being. It's your internal/external organs
and systems, and the actions you perform while on this earth. This part
of the road is where I have spent most of my time helping people. I
believed our health depended solely on our physical body for over 40
years. Even my professional title as a physical therapist was the focus of
all my studies. I believe God called me into the field of physical therapy
when I was a junior in high school. I know His hand was in it from the
beginning. It was also here on my journey I took the first Ex-it off the
"normal" road and made some healthy lifestyle changes.

We have this wonderful physical body; it is a miraculous temple that
houses our spiritual and emotional being. One day I will leave my physical body, but until then there are hundreds of reasons to take care of
the body created for me.

How often do you stop and think about the fact your body and your life here on earth is a gift?

I often hear women say they feel "self-care is selfish"—it's only thinking of oneself. Or some say it is something special for those who are rich and famous. I get it, I once held that same limiting belief, until I was riding in the back of an ambulance. I now believe it is our responsibility as adult human beings to take the time and energy to care for our own bodies. When we care for our body, we are glorifying our creator, we are setting an example to others, and it gives us the energy to live out our purpose.

When we choose not to follow a healthy lifestyle, not to exercise, not to practice self-control, not to get enough sleep, not to drink enough water, not to eat in a healthy manner, or not to care about our own body, we are choosing not to honor God.

"Do you not know that you are God's temple and that God's Spirit dwells in you?"
1 CORINTHIANS 3:16 (ESV)

I believe God will use us for His glory, no matter our circumstances or our health. But, as a follower of Christ, I want to be His hands and feet and it's hard to get through a day when I'm overwhelmed with stress, have no energy, and burdened with dis-ease.

When we are a healthy, willing vessel, God can use us powerfully. You never know what God will call you to do or where He will call you to go. Being prepared spiritually and emotionally is important, but adding in a healthy physical body is giving the Lord the best YOU possible.

As we have we walked this road from the center of the SEP Circle, beginning with the inner circle—your spiritual being and making our way through the emotional connection to your physical being—I hope you can see all of YOU. Each ring of this circle can be thin and delicate, or it can be thick and strong, dependent on you taking care of yourself spiritually, emotionally, and physically. As we walk through the physical being, it will lead us to the next chapter of essentials, which are layers you can add to your circle—much like the bark on a tree to protect you from the outside world and to weather the storms that will come your way. Your physical body must be healthy enough to carry out the actions to get you to the results you desire.

Here is the thing, if in the past you made changes with your physical body and found yourself right back where you were before exercise, changing your diet, or any of the other self-care habits that improve health I want you to know I understand. I've been there.

Western Medicine has taught healthcare from the bottom-up approach (more of a reductionist approach) for years. They start with the symptom and make forced changes—such as a diet or an exercise program or following a doctor's prescription to change the body. If you do it long enough, you will have physical changes occur—weight loss, improved blood sugar, blood pressure, less stress. However, if YOU haven't changed, you find when the diet is over, the exercise program stops, or the prescription runs out that you are right back where you were before—on the "normal" road.

Most Functional Medicine doctors, naturopaths, and health and wellness educators consider themselves going from a top-down approach (more of a holistic approach) where they look at the big picture regarding health and finding the cause instead of just treating the symptoms.

When the Lord gave me the ExSEPshNL Formula, I didn't realize in the beginning that the order was of importance and could make the process faster and with less resistance. With time and lots of failures (what I now know were steps of faith and teaching moments), the order is part of the beauty of the ExSEPshNL Formula.

A popular author, Simon Sinek has what he calls the "Golden Circle" in his book *Start with Why*.[1] Now I haven't read the book, but I watched a TEDx[2] video where he was sharing this concept, and I laughed when I saw it because I realized it's much like my SEP Circle. He's just coming from a business perspective.

SEP Circle = YOU

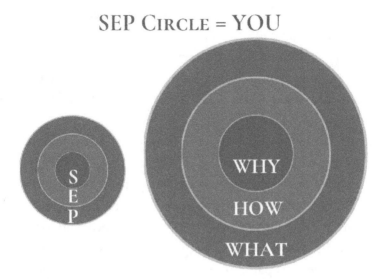

Each ring of this circle can be thin and delicate, or it can be thick and strong, dependent on you taking care of yourself spiritually, emotionally, and physically.

The inner-circle—the Why. The second ring—the How, and the third ring—the What. He shares most people have an outside-in approach to business. They start with the "What" and move towards the "Why," because "what" is the easiest and seen most clearly. The "why" can be a little fuzzy—because as Simon Sinek says, "Why is your purpose, your cause, your belief." Sounds like our Spiritual being to me. If we want genuine change, we must come from an inside-out approach. What I found even more interesting from his video is when he shared it's not based on business philosophy but on biology—biology of the brain.

I promise to tell you how the brain fits into the equation, but right now as we walk through the physical body—I want you to remember what you learned about your spiritual core and think about "why" you want to be healthy and well. Remember the vision challenge? You wrote what you have always dreamed of having, doing what you have always wanted to accomplish, going to the places you have always wanted to go... picturing yourself as the person you were born to be. That is often a snapshot of your WHY.

Think about why loving yourself unconditionally is so important to your health. When you live in a place of unconditional love, there is no need for "I should have done this" or "I should do this"—I want you to let go of the judgment and the shame of the should's as we discuss the physical body. I want you to think about now and tomorrow and love yourself without putting conditions on yourself.

Remember how we moved to the Emotional Connection; this is the "how." How you feel, the driver of your belief. If you find there is something getting between your vision and doing the "what" to get there, it's often right here where we find an emotional blocker. A current emotion created from your beliefs and thoughts, or a trapped emotion from the past. Remember how important forgiveness is to your health? Again, as I lead you down this path, forgive yourself for any past choices or current issues your body may have lingering within.

This chapter in the roadmap is to help you know your body better and lead you towards the "what"—the result you desire—a new beginning, a way to answer the question, "Now *what* do I do?" The ExSEPshNL Formula will guide you from the inside-out as you continue to become the WHO you were created to be.

GUT

"All disease begins in the gut."
~ Hippocrates

One of the first questions I hear when it comes to the health of our body is: *Where do I start?* That's a great question, and one I asked myself when writing this book. I decided to take the advice given over 2,000 years ago, since Hippocrates seemed to have it all figured out—all disease begins in the gut. *Where then does health begin?* This is a question I have spent the last ten years asking myself and learning more and more about, and each time it leads me to the gut. I am now even seeing mainstream doctors learning from Functional Medicine doctors and naturopaths on how the gut affects our health. Often this change occurs after they or a family member have an issue that modern medicine says is incurable or must require long-term medication with dozens of side-effects. Like me, they say enough is enough and look at lifestyle choices to bring health to the body.

So what is our gut? Our gut is our digestive system. This system comprises several organs that include the mouth, esophagus, stomach, small and large intestines—and form a long tube called the gastrointestinal (GI) tract—and ends when we expel waste. Our food moves through the GI tract where it digests, absorbs nutrients, and excretes waste; the pancreas, liver, and gallbladder all produce enzymes, hormones, and other substances needed for digestion to work. When foods can properly process within our gut, we are at our healthiest state.

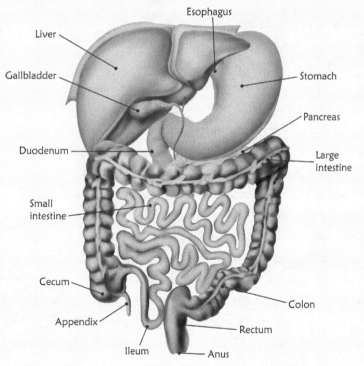

Gastrointestinal tract

Esophagus

Liver

Gallbladder

Stomach

Pancreas

Duodenum

Large intestine

Small intestine

Cecum

Colon

Appendix

Rectum

Ileum

Anus

Did you know your gut has three functions?

1. Digestion of food to produce nutrients for energy.
2. Enteric nervous system- controls motor functions, local blood flow, mucosal transport, and secretions, and modulates immune and endocrine functions.
3. The home of our microbiome where microorganisms that outnumber our own human cells 10:1 flourish.

Most chronic health problems and weight gain lead back to the gut, it only makes sense to start at the gut if you want to improve your health.

Do you have an optimal digestive system or an unhealthy gut?

I know this is often an uncomfortable road to go down. A hard question to ask ourselves. Let me help you. If you are dealing with any of these issues: autoimmune diseases—rheumatoid arthritis, lupus, chronic fatigue syndrome; skin issues—acne, eczema, rosacea; mental health issues—anxiety, depression; metabolic issues—insulin resistance, pre-diabetes, diabetes; gut issues—acid reflux, constipation, diarrhea, and/or obesity it's like you are carrying a big walking billboard with the words—UNHEALTHY GUT.

Yet, many of us have dealt with many of these issues and never knew our gut was unhealthy or played a part in the disease process?

Maybe you are one of the lucky ones and you haven't been diagnosed with a disease—you just deal with headaches, migraines, hormone imbalance, and undiagnosable pain. Oh, maybe that's not lucky. Maybe you want the diagnosis, something to explain how bad you feel. I know that was what I was searching for—an answer, a quick fix, something to take away the pain. No matter what your ailment, modern medicine thinks it has the perfect answer—medication to manage it. Medication does not heal or cure. True healing occurs when we create health.

If you have any of the issues I listed, you might think—*now what?* First, let me say you are not alone. I too walked this road, and I know how our Standard American Diet (SAD) puts us at risk of having gut issues. Let the signs of dis-ease be a sign you need to work on a few wellness strategies targeting your gut.

If your digestive system is not working to break down food, you may have a vitamin and/or mineral deficiency. This is necessary for the body to burn fat and create energy. Studies show micronutrient deficiency can cause as much as an 80% increase in the likelihood of becoming overweight. This means being overweight could be more about malnutrition than overeating. Sounds odd, I know, but have you ever thought maybe the body holds onto fat because it needs to be nourished? It's time to love your gut.

LEAKY GUT

"All disease begins in the leaky gut."
~ Alessio Fasano

Did you know if your gut is not digesting your food it can "leak" into your bloodstream and cause your blood sugar levels to spike, weight gain, and other health issues?[3] Have you heard the popular term going around these days called "leaky gut?"

What is leaky gut? Think of your gut linings like a cheesecloth or a tea towel, it is a tight, thin barrier designed to only let nutrients from well-digested food move through the wall into the bloodstream. If the gut wall is compromised and there are tears or openings that allow food particles (proteins) to leak through the walls of the intestines and into the bloodstream, you have a leaky gut.

What causes tears or openings in the gut lining? When food isn't moving through the gut, fermentation occurs—think rotten, putrefied food sitting there for days. It's kind of like never taking out the trash, it begins to stink and breakdown the trash bag. Food sitting in the gut affects the lining in the same way, and over time causes damage. As these tears or holes appear they allow partially digested food, toxins, and bugs that are in the gut to penetrate and move into the bloodstream. Since they do not belong in the bloodstream, they appear to be foreign invaders to the immune system. Your immune system then attacks the invaders and creates antibodies. This triggers inflammation and changes in the microbiome, slowing down how the gut functions, including fat burning. This is also what makes you swollen and bloated. If you ever have a food panel sensitivity test and pretty much everything you eat comes up—it's because all those foods have not broken down and have leaked through your gut into your bloodstream and are now dangerous to your body. Therefore, even healthy foods can be a problem because food particles don't belong in the bloodstream.

What causes food not to move through the gut? There are several scenarios. Emotional stress can play a big part in not being able to break down food. We cannot be in both the fight, flight, or freeze mode and in the rest and digest mode. We need the parasympathetic system to be engaged for food to digest properly. From a physical standpoint, we need enzymes to breakdown our food and water to move it through. If there is an issue anywhere between the mouth and the small intestine on breaking down the food and moving it through, this can cause an issue in the gut lining. The gut microbiome also plays a part in the breakdown of foods and allowing them to move through. When the microbiome is compromised from excessive drinking, use of NSAIDs, antibiotics, steroids, poor food choices, or a moderate amount of sugar, this can slow down the breakdown of food and cause fermentation and damage to the gut wall.

The good news, just like when cleaning up your house and taking out the trash—the stink goes with it. Our gut is the most highly regenerative organ, and the lining regenerates every five to seven days. When we can give the body what it needs to heal, we can stop the gut from leaking.

What can you do to help improve your gut? First, you must start the rest, digest, and healing process. No worries, I'll share with you a few simple ways to do just that here in the book. Second, walk 30 minutes a day. I know I am sounding like a broken record, but it is one of the easiest ways to support your body—even the gut. Walking or increasing activity stimulates the contractions of the intestines and reduces constipation and studies showed to play an even bigger role than number three, which is a healthy diet to improve your gut health and even reverse disease.

Remember, there is more to your gut than just the place you digest your food—I would like to share with you another function your gut has that I find very interesting. Ready? It's called the Gut-Brain Connection.

GUT-BRAIN CONNECTION

"Anything that affects the gut always affects the brain".
~ Dr. Charles Major

As we started walking down this road, I contemplated where to start. I mean, in some ways it made sense to start at the top—our brain. But did you know that you have two brains? That's where it got complicated and I started with your 'second brain' the one living in your intestinal wall—the gut. Remember the last time you were about to take a test or speak in front of a crowd, go on a first date... You may have experienced butterflies, knots in your stomach, or a sense of unease in your gut. You might have even felt as if you needed to throw up. I've been there!

Those sensations are more than just minor feelings. That's a sign of your gut communicating with your brain and vice versa. And when your gut is in a state of dysfunction, your body shows symptoms such as brain fog, mood swings, anxiety, and even depression. Multiple studies on the gut-brain connection have shown that an imbalance in your microbiome within your gut can affect your brain. It is revolutionizing the way medicine looks at mental health disorders and their treatments.

You have what we call the enteric nervous system within your gut, and it shares many of the same features as the brain in your head. It even influences behavior and sends messages by the vagus nerve to your brain upstairs. You have 500 million neurons lining your gut, over 40 different known neurotransmitters being created—50 percent of dopamine is created in both the brain upstairs and downstairs, however, serotonin "happy molecule" only 5 percent is created upstairs and 95 percent is created in the gut. When we take care of our gut, we are happy. When we don't—we don't feel good. Over 90 percent of the fibers in the vagus nerve go from the gut to the brain, and less than 10 percent go from the brain to the gut. So if the gut is doing most of the communicating, who is in control—head brain or gut brain?

Each of our brains has different functions—let's call the head brain #1 since that's what we think of as our brain and the gut we will call brain #2.

Brain #1 is where we learn—it's our logical brain and where we make a lot of our decisions. But let's spend some time with brain #2. Have you heard of "Gut Feelings?" A gut feeling is an instinct (natural behavior) or intuition (immediate feeling—6th sense). You know when you say something such as, "I had a feeling that was going to happen." We know something without knowing why we know it—that feeling comes from the gut. Some believe that intuition is a gift from God. Research has shown our past traumas strengthen our intuition. The question is: Should you trust brain #1 or brain #2 when making a decision?

I cannot tell you how many times my gut has told me something about someone or something, and I have no proof—others don't agree and years later find out—I was right. I agree past traumas can strengthen our gut instincts. So how do we make our decisions?

Brain #1 uses logic and emotion—the knowledge you have learned and the models you have created from your beliefs and your emotions; you then process the information and come up with a decision.

Brain #2 uses intuition—and gives you an instant first warning sign to help with your decision. Often, if you wait for brain #1 to decide, you may wait a long time—especially if you don't already have the knowledge.

A better question may even be: Does your gut seem to be consistently right? If so, listen to it. It may even save your life. People have awakened in the middle of the night and had this gut feeling (protective instinct) something was wrong and left the house—only to find a few minutes later that there was a gas explosion. If they had waited until the fire alarm went off or found the gas leak, it would have been too late.

I said "no" to antidepressants based on my gut feelings. Then I researched to see if I could find why I should or shouldn't take them. I found a few things, and it spurred me to keep looking—this was one reason I went to the naturopath. Years later, after having genetic testing, I learned a lot of my gut feelings fit with the results my genetic profile showed. I am not a good genetic match up for several drugs, and antidepressants are one of them.

Are you listening to your gut instinct that often feels like butterflies (physiological stress response), nausea (increased hormones), or even an upset stomach (less blood and/or digestive juices in the stomach)? Or are you ignoring those feelings or covering up your emotions with drugs or even food? Studies have shown medications may prevent you from listening to your gut—both the physical signs and the emotional signs that could give you the answers you need for true healing.

So as I learned all about the Gut-Brain connection, I had these questions: If our emotions affect our gut—can our gut affect our emotions? Is depression a gut illness or a mental illness?

When I researched these very questions, I found Dr. Kelly Brogan, MD, and shared with you some of her findings in the previous chapters.[4] She has found that the Brain-Gut are so connected that depression is just a symptom of gut dysfunction. Does that mean we have been treating the wrong brain?

Now, not everyone feels gut symptoms to have gut issues—just like we can stuff our emotions and not even be aware of how they are affecting us—the same goes for our gut. I didn't realize until 2014 my hormonal/emotional issues were rooted in my gut. When I had some gut testing done, I found out I had a moderate amount of candida and lots of different parasites. I was horrified and thought I was the only one until I read the book *Every Body Has Parasites: If You're Alive, You're at Risk!*[5]

And yes, it made me feel better to learn I was not the only one. I didn't "feel" I had gut issues—because I didn't have gut pain. You don't need to have gut pain to have a dysfunctional gut.

What I realized later is when I changed my diet 40 days before my 40th birthday, I was healing my gut, which helped my hormones/emotions. The other changes I had made like no longer taking ibuprofen and stopping the toxic household and beauty care products that were killing my good bacteria allowed my gut to make more happy molecules. How do I know? Because not only did I feel better emotionally and have fewer physical issues, but when I would eat more sugar or be around more toxins, my symptoms would return. I am still a work in progress and I know my gut will need tender loving care for all the abuse received the first 40 years of my life. I am passionate about helping others on this same journey to understand and heal. Our gut problems are related to our own personal choices—food, toxic products, and not lowering our stress.

Before 2012, I believed my hormonal/emotional roller coaster was who I was—it defined me and in some ways it did. With time I realized it was my inability to handle childhood and adulthood traumas and the self-hatred that led me to the choices I made. These choices affected my gut and my emotions. The messages brain #2 would send to brain #1 led to my thoughts, emotions, feelings along with actions and results. But it wasn't just my DNA that was doing the talking. We have a whole microbiome full of bacteria—10 times more bacterial cells in our body than human cells. That looks like about 100 trillion bacterial cells in our body.

Let's look at that bacteria for just a minute. What have we been doing to our gut for years? We have been killing the bacteria within us—antibiotics, environmental products used to clean our water and kill the weeds and the bugs. What is it doing to our bacteria? What is it doing to us?

We have this exceptional microbiome within our gut. Just imagine with me for a moment that this microbiome is your own little community. You can feed your community the right foods and give them the right environment and stay balanced and happy. Or you can feed your community the wrong products and give them the wrong environment and be out of balance and depressed. Whichever choice you make affects not only your gut, but the messages it sends to your brain.,

Bacteria is in direct communication with our enteric nervous system—our brain #2. Researchers have connected specific bacteria to those who are more anxious and/or depressed.[6] What about those sugar addictions—could it be the bacteria begging for more? Research has shown that certain foods and supplements such as probiotics can help with anxiety and depression. Our bacteria matter.

I shared with you my White Flour Tortilla story, and the last thing I ever wanted to do was yell at my kids. So how did that one white flour tortilla send me over the edge? I believe what I fed my bacteria sent a message to both of my brains. This was not a relaxing, calm kind of message, this was a message of anger that I took out on those I loved most. No, this is not to blame them (my kids or my bacteria)—I was in control, I chose what the bacteria ate, and it was now clear to me both my brains had a reaction to that white flour tortilla. Now it was my time to take responsibility.

What messages are your bacteria sending to your brain?

BRAIN- HEART- GUT CONNECTION

"It seems both heart and gut have a mind of their own and when they work together harmoniously with the brain then it creates a healthy body, powerful mind and happiness"

~ Anil Rajvanshi

We started at our gut and walked to our brain, but what about the organ between the two we call our heart? Our body is this wonderful creation and the more we learn about some of these wonderful connections between the heart, brain, and gut we also learn keys to our health.

The heart communicates to the brain and gut in four ways:

1. Neurological communication through the nervous system

2. Biochemical communication through hormones and neuro-transmitters

3. Biophysical communication through pulse waves

4. Energetic communication through the electromagnetic field that spans up to 3 feet from the heart

Some even say the "heart" has its own little brain. Again, the heart talks to the brain in our head more than our brain talks to our heart. I believe our heart connects our spiritual, emotional, and physical beings.

I had the opportunity as a physical therapist to watch an open-heart surgery. This was the most amazing and stressful surgery I had ever seen. Not only did I watch them open this man's chest, but I saw them attach him to a bypass machine and witness his heart stop beating. They worked diligently on fixing his heart. His life was in the hands of the doctors and nurses as I stood over his head watching the whole procedure, wondering who this man was, what his life looked like before this surgery, and what had caused his heart disease to begin with. I was young and I remember thinking about what his life would be like after surgery. Then it was the moment we were all waiting for—the surgeon/medical staff to restart the heart. I am pretty sure I was holding my breath in anticipation. The doctor used a little mini paddle to send an electrical signal to restart his heart. Nothing. I prayed. He shocked it again. Nothing. Then the doctor put down the paddle, took the heart in his hand, and thumped it. The heart began to beat and I let out a breath of relief. The room was full of celebration. Whenever I think of the heart, I still picture that heart in the doctor's hand—the organ that decides our fate on this earth between life and death.

The heart is a muscle that pumps blood, but it's also an endocrine gland that secretes hormones. The heart signals the brain in multiple ways and even releases peptides that stimulate the pituitary gland in the brain to release hormones like oxytocin "the love hormone." We then feel wonderful emotions like joy and happiness and maybe even butterflies in our gut.

What connects the brain, heart, and gut? The vagus nerve. Yes, the vagus nerve may be the **key** to a healthy brain, healthy heart, and a healthy gut—a healthier YOU.

You may remember the vagus nerve in the previous chapter. It played a part in our emotional health and also plays a part in our physical health. *Are you curious to know what turns the key to activate the vagus nerve and send calming messages throughout your body?* **Deep breathing.** Yes, this amazing free exercise you can do anytime, anywhere turns the key that stimulates the parasympathetic nervous system to "rest, digest and heal" and has the brain, heart, and gut working together harmoniously to create a healthy body. This amazing self-care habit can improve your mental clarity and focus along with increased creativity while reducing blood pressure, creating optimal rhythm patterns of the heart, helping the gut perform better, and clean out the colon.

How we breathe sends information through the vagus nerve and into the brain to make changes. When we breathe slowly, the heart slows, and we relax. This sends a message to our gut—*time to digest.*

When we breathe quickly, our brain sends a message for our heart to speed up and our gut gets the message to stop digesting and we put healing on hold.

Did you catch that—how you breathe changes your health?
Each exhale triggers the relaxation response. When we hold our breath (stress response) we feel anxious. The most calming way to breathe and keep the key turned to the healing state is to breathe 5 seconds in and 5 seconds out regularly. If we want to turn on the vagus nerve, then a longer exhale will flip the switch.

When I worked in a local hospital, I spent a year working in Cardiac Rehab. I often saw patients go from having heart surgery to our Outpatient Cardiac Rehab program, where we would start patients on a healthy heart regimen of exercises and diet. My job was to teach them deep breathing, a walking program on the treadmill, and strengthening exercises while I hooked them up to a monitor to watch their heart rhythm through the entire process. I loved watching the heartbeat and to see how the actions they performed would change the frequency and rhythm of their heart. It was amazing to watch the progress these patients made when changing the previous lifestyle habits that led them to the hospital. When they graduated from the program, we celebrated with them to continue on their journey. Many continued to workout in our hospital gym and others we would see months later back on the hospital floor. My first question when I would re-evaluate them, "Have you continued with your healthy heart regimen?" Sadly, the answer was "no." I know how hard it is to change lifestyle habits when we do it only from the physical side—when we are following a plan given to us, but no real change has occurred within our heart—our beliefs, our emotions, and the heart walls blocking us from a future of growth and health.

What I have found on my journey is this disconnect—my brain telling me one thing, my heart telling me another, and my gut disagreeing with both of them. It is this overwhelming uncertainty of which way to go, what to do. Can you go down three separate roads at one time? No! Instead you weave back and forth on the highway of life depending on which of the three are in the most control at that very moment.

When you use deep breathing exercises, a connection occurs between the brain, the heart, and the gut, it is like a harmonic symphony—a calmness you feel all over. No longer do you feel the chaos and overwhelm inside. You can then make healthy choices for yourself from a place of knowing and peace. A practice of deep breathing can help anyone achieve less stress that brings holistic health.

ExSEPshNL Solution: Less Stress

GUT-LUNG CONNECTION

"Dysbiosis in gut microbiota has been implicated in several lung diseases, including allergy, asthma and cystic fibrosis."
~ Swadha Anand

Deep breathing requires the ability of the lungs to expand with an inhale and deflate as you exhale. I know many women today who have a hard time breathing because of allergies, asthma, sinus issues, and the list goes on. Just like we have found the gut connected to the brain and the heart, the gut-lung connection plays a big role in our health too. Remember, if our gut microbiome (community) is out of balance, it affects the entire body.

Inside the lining of our nose, cheeks and gut are intestinal mast cells that communicate with our enteric neurons and could be the connection between allergies, our gut, and even our emotions. We often blame pollen from trees for our allergy symptoms, but why does one person appear to be allergic to some things, and another person is not? Now there are a lot of theories out there and a lot more research needed in this area, but I feel what I have learned is important enough for you to think about.

The Johns Hopkins University Research Team from 1996 showed that nothing you breathe causes an asthmatic attack.[7] It can be inherited, but it is coming out of deep-rooted fear, anxiety, and stress. That research was found by our western medical community, what does that mean? To me, it means that our physical issues are connected to our emotions more than we will probably ever understand.

When dealing with allergies most people grab an antihistamine, a popular one is Benadryl, a histamine blocker. Your mast cells have these little receptors, and when something irritates them, they put off histamine. A histamine blocker goes in and blocks these receptors. I don't know about you, but I don't want a drug blocking my body, I want to know why something is irritating it. Why is it the "norm" when we are irritated emotionally or physically we want to block or stop the symptom or emotion and pretend it's not there?

What if instead of a drug we used something more natural? A technique or a tool that supports or works with our body. My choice is often essential oils because I have found they give my body what it needs to balance. Looking at the essential oil lavender from the physiological side, it seems like the perfect fit—a natural antihistamine. But I didn't know if I wanted even something natural stopping my body from doing what it was created to do.

So, I did a little research and found on pubmed.gov how lavender works.[8] See, mast cells in our body attract lavender. I love how God made plants to work with humans. When lavender gets to the mast cells, it does not block the receptors. Do you know what it does instead? It cleans the receptors off. In my mind I see the little scrubbing bubble commercial, cleaning the bathtub, but in this case our receptor sites. So if something irritates the mast cells, doesn't it make sense to clean the body instead of blocking it? That's what lavender does.

What if we started looking at our physical symptoms and started asking, "How can I clean up what's going on instead of blocking and stopping the symptoms?" This is what I hope you learn as we continue to walk and talk. When we ask questions, we find answers to our health instead of more issues. I now look deeper from all sides: spiritual, emotional, and physical, and what I have learned has been amazing. Which led me to the next question.

Could breathing issues have an emotional tie? Henry W. Wright in his book *A More Excellent Way to Be in Health* believes the *fear of abandonment* coupled with *insecurity is the* greatest reason for breathing difficulties.[7]

The essential oil connected to *abandonment* is lavender. Interesting, isn't it? Research has shown for years lavender helps people become more relaxed, even serene and stimulates the vagus nerve.[9] But for some lavender appears to have a negative reaction. We often see this when someone has a trapped emotion. Essential oils have a frequency, and so do the trapped emotions—when a trapped emotion does not want to be released, the oil can cause an irritation. I thought lavender smelled awful for years, and early in the writing of my penny story, I realized I had the trapped emotion: *abandonment*. After years of emotional releases and using lavender, I now love the smell and use it daily.

I was talking to a mom and teenage daughter about essential oils one night, and the mom was looking for something to help her daughter sleep. She had a lot of health issues and the doctors couldn't find the cause. These issues were also affecting her sleep, which was causing her problems with finishing school.

I told her, "lavender helps many people get better sleep." The mom said, "I think she is allergic to lavender." I asked her why and was told she was allergic to a lot of things, but whenever they would diffuse lavender, she would throw up. Throwing up and nausea were the two biggest issues the doctors couldn't find a cause or a cure for this girl. I shared with both the mom and the daughter that often we can have a connection to an oil from an emotional perspective and showed her my *Releasing Emotional Patterns with Essential Oils* book and how *abandonment* is the emotion connected to that oil. The mom quickly said, "I doubt that's the reason—I have never abandoned her." I shared with the mom and daughter that *abandonment* from a child's view and an adult's view may be different and could still cause trauma. I told them the story of my oldest son crying at three years old when he watched videos of himself as a baby—because he was all alone in the videos. Now we were right there, just out of the camera's view, but because he could not see us—he felt like we had *abandoned* the baby—him. The alarm point—where we hold *abandonment* is the *small intestine (aka the gut)*.

I then had a *gut feeling* I needed to go deeper and share my personal story—"I never thought about being *abandoned* until I began learning more about releasing trapped emotions. *Abandonment* could mean the loss of a parent, divorce, or it could be a belief created by a child based on only what they see—not what was necessarily true as with my son. The emotion could even be passed down from the mother if she felt *abandoned* during her pregnancy... when I looked at my past, I realized I carried the trapped emotion *abandonment* by my biological father, who I had never met."

The daughter began crying and said, *"I don't know my biological father either."* Her mom sat up straight and tall, *"but she's never wanted to know him—she has a wonderful family."* The teenage girl slumped down in her chair and said, *"You never ask how I feel."*

How often do we search everywhere for the answers to physical symptoms, but we never ask the person or ourselves what we are feeling?

I asked if I could show her how to release the trapped emotion of *abandonment,* and she and her mother were willing. Even though I think we were all a little apprehensive that she might throw up—we had a trash can nearby. We went through the process and a few weeks later I received an email from the mom thanking me. She and her daughter had talked, and she was no longer throwing up when they diffused lavender and she was sleeping better.

It's stories like that one that gives me the strength to share this information with you—to walk with you on this journey with the ExSEPshNL Formula leading us through our magnificent physical being.

**Go to www.shawnacale.com/book-bonus
Printable Journal Pages and Bonus Resources
to Live an Exceptional Life.**

ACTION: USE LAVENDER ESSENTIAL OIL

1. Do you have breathing or lung issues? Do you have gut issues? Do you have anxiety or stress? Do you have sleeping issues? Could you be holding onto the emotion of *abandonment* or *insecurity* in your life? Use the *Releasing Emotional Patterns with Essential Oils*[10] book using lavender[11] and begin the healing process.

IMMUNE SYSTEM

"Every act of kindness on your part is a boost to your own immune system."
~ Marianne Williamson

As we continue to walk this road that leads to health, I want to share with you the importance of your immune system. It's an amazing network of cells and proteins that protect your body from toxic substances, illness, and disease. Did you know you have two lines of defense? They call the first one the innate immune system and it has an immediate response time and lasts up to 96 hours. Its first job is to clean up: it gets rid of all bacteria and viruses that cause disease. Then the mast cells and dendritic cells bring in the second line of defense if needed.

This second line of defense is called the adaptive immune system, and it comes into play about 96 hours after the innate and only called in if it has found a foreign invader. This includes lymphocytes: T cells (the communicators) and B cells that produce an antibody for a specific invader. It then keeps a record of every foreign invader it has ever defeated so it can recognize and destroy it if it enters the body again. This includes bacteria, viruses, fungi, parasites, undigested food particles, or unhealthy cells such as cancer cells. Your immune system includes your white blood cells, bone marrow, antibodies, thymus, spleen, liver, skin, lungs, lymphatic system, and 70 percent or more of the immune system is in the gut. My goal is to share a fresh perspective on how the immune system works and how it plays a part in the disease process.

In the past, when my body was not working the way I would like—let's use the example of a runny nose—I would get mad at my body. I would think, *Now I am sick—why isn't my immune system taking care of me, why is my body betraying me?*

Guess what? It was doing what God created it to do. Snot is how the body gets rid of the toxins from within. When I would do things to stop it, I wasn't allowing my immune system to do its job. Now, I do my best to be kind to myself and thank my immune system for letting go of the toxins and doing an amazing job of healing. I know it may sound silly but I rarely get a runny nose and if I do—I help my body release the snot, thank it, and move on.

A fever is when the body temperature rises, which happens when we get an infection or a virus. This again is an immune system response. It is your body killing the invaders and triggering the body's repair process. Instead of fighting it, I have induced a low-grade fever with a nice hot bath with Epsom salt and ginger or clove essential oil to raise my body temperature and help support my immune system by getting rid of those yucky invaders. I can't remember the last time I felt bad for over 12-24 hours.

Did you know your cells have a health cycle? During this cycle, if your cell has any type of threat (stressor)—trauma, infection, virus, parasite it turns on the cell danger response—the mitochondria within the cell flips a switch to begin the repair process your body needs for healing also known as acute inflammation.[12]

Cell Danger Response

Stage 1: The cell walls itself off from the rest of the body to protect itself from further infection, illness, or injury. You can typically see it and/or feel it and it includes—pain, redness, immobility, swelling, and heat. The neurotransmitter histamine plays a part in this process and recruits the immune response—to neutralize the area (independent from the rest of the body). It lasts a few minutes to a few days. This is a good thing. It is the body doing its job and protecting the rest of your body.

Stage 2: This is the repair and rebuild stage. Often we just need to be gentle and kind to our body and let it go through this healing process.

Stage 3: Cells reconnect to the health cycle and turn down the immune system—the vagus nerve is the switch that turns off the inflammation.

Do you think it's a good idea to stop any of those three stages?

How often do we do everything we can to block the healing stage so we can carry on as if nothing happened? I am no different from you; I don't want to feel sick or be sick. I want to feel great all the time. But are we causing more illness than health when stopping the body from doing what it was created to do?

In my house, we have found amazing ways to support our body and immune system as it is going through the cell danger response and one of our favorites is the Raindrop Technique that I learned back in 2012. It uses some wonderful essential oils like oregano, thyme, marjoram, basil, cypress, wintergreen, and peppermint. These essential oils all work at the cellular level to help the body through the healing process. When we give our body a little tender loving care, it repays us with health and well-being.

Why does acute inflammation go chronic, and what can we do about it? When cells are stuck in a repeating loop through the three stages, it is because the cell still believes it is in danger and acute inflammation becomes chronic inflammation. This leads to long-term suffering and chronic disease. Today our bodies are overloaded with stressors and/or ACEs (Adverse Childhood Experiences) that cause the body to be in the fight, flight, or freeze state and the cells get stuck in the cell danger response.

Could you have cells stuck in the cell danger response?

- Do you have body pain, especially in the joints?
- Do you have skin rashes, such as eczema or psoriasis?
- Do you have excessive mucus production (ie, always needing to clear your throat or blow your nose)?
- Do you have low energy, despite sufficient sleep?
- Do you have poor digestion, including bloating, abdominal pain, constipation, and/or loose stools?

If you said yes to even one of those, you may have chronic inflammation in your body. Believe me, you are not alone, 60 percent of the

American population have cells stuck in this loop. Yes, this sounds a lot like a "leaky gut" because those cells in the lining are in the cell danger response.

Understanding chronic inflammation is critical. We know this inflammation as the "Silent Killer" and it occurs inside the body without noticeable signs like acute inflammation. The person may complain they don't feel good for years. Then one day diagnosed with a disease. As if it just magically appeared or happened overnight. It's not because the doctor missed the disease—it's because it was still in the beginning stages, often known as "inflammation" and wasn't at the disease state yet.

Let's dive into what a disease is? A disease is a set of symptoms: a list of signs that have been grouped together and given a name. If you want to feel better, don't wait to have all the symptoms and receive the name of a disease to make changes. Start making changes now and beat the disease.

As I have said before, I was on the road that led to disease. I had all the signs of chronic inflammation in my early 20s. I knew this from what I had learned in physical therapy school, but what I had not been taught was lifestyle habits were the cause, and lifestyle habits were the solution.

One way to check to see what the levels of inflammation are in your body is to have your CRP (C-reactive protein) checked, the liver makes this protein, and it gives you an idea of where you are at regarding your own health.

If your CRP is not at its optimal level (women under 1.0 mg/L) but closer to the 10.0 mg/L your doctor will do more tests to see if the chronic inflammation has led to a disease like Alzheimer's, arthritis, an autoimmune disease, cancer, cardiovascular disease, diabetes, fatty liver disease. But there is a lot of inflammatory destruction that can go on between 1.0 -10.0 mg/L. Only when the mitochondria within the cells believe it is safe will the healing be completed. The key to decreasing chronic inflammation and preventing disease is good vagal tone and flipping the inflammation switch off with the vagus nerve.

When I learned the secret to how the immune system switches off the inflammatory response at the perfect time, I was excited. Resolvents are the key, not medications. They are simply fatty acids, which are the building blocks of the fat in our bodies and the food we eat. Did I just say fat? Yes! During digestion, the body breaks down fats into fatty acids, which absorb into the bloodstream and increases vagal tone. This stimulates the vagus nerve by flipping the switch to reconnect the cells from the cell danger response to the health cycle. One of the most essential resolvents is Omega 3's, and that is why they are so important to our health. They support the natural progression of the inflammatory process instead of stopping or blocking the process from doing its job.

Go to www.shawnacale.com/book-bonus
Printable Journal Pages and Bonus Resources
to Live an Exceptional Life.

ACTION: RESET VAGUS NERVE

1. Walking 20-30 minutes per day increases vagal tone and decreases chronic inflammation.

2. The practice of gratitude, unconditional love, and forgiveness resets the vagus nerve and allows the cells to feel safe and move into the health cycle.

3. Deep Breathing exercises stimulate the vagus nerve and allow the cell danger response to complete the three stages.

4. Increase Omega-3 Fatty Acids (resolvents) to your daily diet to stimulate the vagus nerve and flip the switch from the cell danger response to the health cycle. Fatty fish, walnuts, pecans, chia seeds, flax seeds, Brussels sprouts, and avocados are some of my daily favorites.

LIVER

"Whenever the brain and heart fight it is always the liver that suffers."
~ Unknown

Let me tell you about what I lovingly call the "mom" of the human body. She's your liver and plays a role in your immune system and gives you a clue on the state of inflammation in your body. She is the largest internal organ and stays busy taking care of over 500 biological processes. She fights infection; neutralizes toxins, breaks down nutrients, stores nutrients, produces amino acids, produces hormones, helps make blood, balances blood sugar, regulates blood pressure, supports thyroid health. Your liver affects every organ and system. You will feel it if she does not show up and do her job. *How does she do all those things?* She filters everything that enters your body, including every toxin—and we live in a toxic world. Remember, your emotions are toxic too—and anger is the toxic emotion that likes to hang out in your liver.

If the liver has too much work to do, it becomes sluggish and you see more issues—gut issues and high blood pressure are just a few. Most of us want to be healthy? I thought I was making excellent choices, but metabolic health and inflammation are a two-way highway. I liked my sugar, and the lack of fat in my diet brought on insulin resistance. Now, this wasn't anything a doctor told me, but after years of reading the signs and symptoms, I asked for blood work to see my metabolic panel. The symptoms were not lying. My blood cells had become resistant to insulin. You know how after a while kids yelling and screaming or the TV being up loud becomes the "norm" and you just start ignoring it. Our body does the same thing. It stops allowing the insulin in—which carries the glucose to the cells for energy and this leaves more glucose in the blood, which tells the pancreas to make more insulin, which drives inflammation and with time Type 2 diabetes. The liver and fat cells then store the extra glucose, and too much glucose will cause fatty liver.

How do you know if you have a fatty or sluggish liver?

- Elevated "LDL" cholesterol
- Elevated Triglycerides
- Reduced "HDL" cholesterol
- Weight gain
- Heart disease
- Digestive problems
- Skin issues
- Hormonal imbalance
- Blood sugar imbalance
- Swollen feet
- Body odor
- Bad breath
- Fatigue
- Nausea

For years I dealt with a sluggish liver (based on my symptoms) and never knew it. I would complain of feeling nauseated in the mornings, issues with weight gain, skin issues like acne, and hormonal imbalances. I did not understand the toxins I was putting in my body and on my body were causing my "mom" inside to be worn-out and tired, which made me as a mom feel the same way, overwhelmed and done.

What I have learned through the past 10 years is supporting my liver daily is true self-care for my internal "mom" because less stress on my body, less anger, less pain, and more energy gives me more time to be the mom I was created to be.

Here's some more good news: Your liver can regenerate with as little as 25 percent of the original liver mass to its full size! You can re-new your liver with the right choices (self-care). When you love your liver—your "mom" is no longer tired and sluggish!

Go to www.shawnacale.com/book-bonus
Printable Journal Pages and Bonus Resources
to Live an Exceptional Life.

ACTION: LOVE YOUR LIVER

1. Walking is key to a healthy liver by decreasing stress on the liver and increasing energy levels.

2. Choosing natural cleaning and beauty care products will decrease the toxic load on your liver.

3. Drinking filtered water with lemon juice or lemon essential oil to help cleanse your liver.

4. Coffee Enemas are one of the fastest and most economical ways to detoxify your liver.[18]

CHRONIC INFLAMMATION

"Inflammation is in the background of every single major illness."
~Julie Daniluk

I have taken you to see the gut, the brain, the heart, the lungs, and the liver. We can see how chronic inflammation in one area can trickle down to other organs and systems.

I believe Alzheimer's to be an inflammatory disease. The question is, what has caused the inflammation in the first place? Is there an infection in the brain responding to some foreign microorganism? An inflamed brain affects one's memory and ability to recall. Many women believe their scattered thoughts and trouble focusing are just a part of aging—but they're not. They are a sign of silent inflammation.

I have watched family members and patients with this awful disease, and I have seen how it affects those they love. Knowing chronic inflammation is a sign that keeps me diligent in listening and understanding when my body is inflamed and what I can do to turn off the inflammation. It has also been called Type III Diabetes.[15]

Chronic inflammation is also a major cause of autoimmune diseases. I believe there are several reasons inflammation can occur. One mechanism being researched is genetic vulnerability. Certain genes (DNA that make proteins) often look like proteins specific bacteria make. Our immune system will see (new) bacteria as a foreign invader and make an antibody to protect us. Anytime it sees this protein now, it will take care of it. The problem begins when our immune system sees a similar protein (our own) and thinks it could be dangerous too—we know this as molecular mimicry, and once this happens an autoimmune disease is born. They are finding with more and more autoimmune diseases, there was a specific infection that started the process, and often there is a genetic link that caused the body to fight itself.

Another mechanism is when food appears to cause autoimmune disease. We often have genes that make proteins that look similar to the proteins in certain foods—wheat, tomatoes, soy are some of the most common, the immune system gets confused. When the body makes antibodies to proteins in wheat, your body is trying to protect you from what it thinks is danger again because of this molecular mimicry, but it fights your own proteins too. Often these proteins line the joints of the body.

Remember your immune system also lies in your gut and when it is not working, it allows larger particles (proteins) into your bloodstream (leaky gut). Your immune system thinks they are invaders and attacks and the antibodies then find their way to attacking other healthy cells in your body. This is your body at war with itself.

Research has linked cancer to chronic inflammation because tumors are where inflammation was once present. Again, the question often is why is there inflammation in the first place?

This same chronic inflammation triggers increased production of cholesterol as the body attempts to repair the lining of blood vessels and arteries from damage, often causing a build-up and cardiovascular disease.

Today heart disease is the leading cause of death for women and is known as the "Silent Killer." Isn't that what I said they call chronic inflammation? Why do some call hypertension (high blood pressure) the "Silent Killer" too? These are all related—chronic inflammation leads to hypertension which leads to heart disease, and all three lead to death.

Studies show those with depression to have 30 percent more inflammation in the brain and gut due to certain microorganisms found in the gut.[6] Musculoskeletal pain is another sign of chronic inflammation and is a big component of osteoarthritis. The disease doctors said for years was just wear and tear from old age. I have seen girls as young as thirteen have osteoarthritis the age of an 80-year-old. This is no longer an old age issue. This is a chronic inflammation issue.

Inflammation causes common everyday aches and pains in joints and muscles. If your body feels sore and stiff, systemic inflammation is likely to be the problem.

I believe this was the road I was traveling with my own joint pain in my legs and shoulders as a young child until I was forty years old. I took ibuprofen daily for headaches, joint pain, cramps, all signs of chronic inflammation. I knew it was inflammation and knew the damage inflammation caused, so when I asked a doctor when I was in my 20s what to do—he told me to take ibuprofen as the bottle suggested until it no longer worked for me, and then I would need to move up to a prescription.

Here's the thing: I was taking a drug to block/hide my symptoms. Eventually, I realized I was not taking care of the problem. The cause was affecting damage in other areas, and the road I was traveling was leading me to a list of diseases like autoimmune disorders—rheumatoid arthritis, diabetes, and heart disease. It would only make sense if it was an issue of getting older that I would have more joint pain and issues today than I did 10 years ago, but with the changes in my diet and with other stressors being removed my immune system is working for me and not against me.

I want better for you. I want you to know and understand what you can do to improve your health so you can live the life you desire without health issues blocking you from the exceptional life.

When I started self-care habits, lifestyle changes to improve my health, my inflammation decreased and my symptoms disappeared. I have not had one ibuprofen since May 2011 and I have fewer headaches, joint pain, cramps than I had in my teens.

You don't have to live with chronic inflammation. You simply have to make changes to allow your body to heal.

LYMPHATIC SYSTEM

"Love your lymphatics, they're the only ones you've got!"
~ Sue Callison

Have you ever wondered if inflammation is part of our immune system and our immune system's job is to fight disease, why is it causing so much havoc to our bodies? Often it's because our lymphatic system, a part of our immune system crucial for keeping fluid levels in balance and for protecting us from infections, bacteria, cancers, inflammation, and other potential threats, is not doing its job.

Keeping your lymphatic flow free from congestion is critical to your health and well-being. It is a network of lymphatic vessels, lymph nodes, and blood vessels, that work to carry fluids from your tissues to your blood and vice versa. You also have GALT—Gut Associated Lymphatic Tissues in the digestive system to protect invasions in the gut.

I like to think of the lymphatic system as the body's sewage system. It carries lymph—a clear watery fluid along with protein molecules, glucose, salt, and other substances found on their way. Within your lymphatic system, you have little valves that ensure it carries fluid in the right direction and towards lymph organs such as the adenoids, tonsils, thymus, spleen, and lymph nodes. Most lymph nodes are in the throat, armpits, chest, abdomen, and groin. Their job is to fight infections, help you recover from illness, and heal wounds with the use of infection-fighting white blood cells—also known as lymphocytes.

When you come into contact with bacteria, toxins, microbes and they find their way to the lymphatic system, these organisms are trapped and your immune system does its job to attack and destroy them. Once destroyed, they go back into the blood system through the lymph nodes. When your lymph system is healthy and well-functioning, you won't even know that it's doing its job.

However, if your lymphatic system is congested and unable to do its job and you find your body is experiencing abnormal water retention, painful swelling (often seen as bloating, puffiness, and overall run-down feeling) this is a sign your body is fighting chronic infections. It could be an issue in the gut creating your sewage system to stop up and cause more havoc in the body by allowing chronic inflammation to continue because of the lack of normal detoxification and removal of toxins necessary for your body to be healthy. (Remember when the trash isn't taken out, it causes issues.)

What causes the lymphatic system within the immune system to go awry? Well, like most things, we find certain lifestyle factors—daily ones that are promoting ongoing inflammation. Want to guess the #1?

If you guessed stress, you were correct. It can also lead to lymph congestion. When your body is under stress, it creates stress-fighting hormones which lead to a variety of health issues. It then affects our ability to fight infections, digest, maintain a healthy hormone balance... and the list goes on. In fact, studies find at least 80 percent of autoimmune diseases follow a time of high emotional stress.[16] One of the first things you can do to help treat any of these inflammatory processes is to get your stress under control.

What's one of the best ways to decrease inflammation and get the lymphatic system moving? I'll give you a hint—it's a four-letter word.

If you guessed—walk, you're right! Stress is telling our body something is wrong—like a bear is chasing us. If a bear is chasing us, we need to get away. When we walk, our body sends signals saying we are moving to safety. When we are safe, our vagus nerve tells our digestive system to turn back on and digest our food, which gives us the energy we need to continue through the day.

When you are not moving the lymphatic system gets congested, your body gets stiff and your body thinks there is an actual injury (cell danger response) so it sends white blood cells to fix the area—but the only problem was lack of movement. Then you hurt so you move less and the chronic condition continues on and before you know it you are diagnosed with any of several diseases, all from chronic inflammation that could have been prevented.

Remember walking 30 minutes a day has been proven to bring down chronic inflammation and one reason as a physical therapist my goal was always to get patients walking ASAP.

A lack of physical activity also slows down the lymph fluid from moving because it relies on breathing and pressure from muscle movement. Lacking this pressure, because of too much sitting, causes a congested lymph system too.

Deep breathing activates the vagus nerve, helps decrease stress, and also encourages the contraction and relaxation of the muscles in the chest. Your rib cage is a major lymphatic pump necessary for healthy lymphatic flow. So just like walking is important to help push toxins out of your body and to decrease the chance of debris building up. Deep breathing promotes intrathoracic pressure and allows your lungs to press fluid back into your bloodstream and improve oxygen to your cells and proper lymph movement and detoxification.

PHYSICAL STRESS

"Stress is the ability to decide what's important."
~ Unknown

There is so much to our physical body—cells, tissues, organs, systems that all work together to allow us to think, move, live. Each choice we make plays a part in how our body can respond to daily life. Physical stressors can strengthen us or knock us down.

Physical stress is any trauma to the body (injury, infection, or surgery). Intense exercise, physical labor, and over-exertion are also forms of physical stress. Even environmental pollution (pesticides, herbicides, toxins, heavy metals, lack of light, radiation, noise, electromagnetic fields) all can cause physical stress to the body. Inadequate oxygen, low/high blood sugar, hormonal/neurotransmitter imbalances, dietary stress (nutritional deficiencies, food allergies, sensitivities, unhealthy eating habits) all-cause physical stress. Substance abuse, dental challenges, musculoskeletal misalignments/imbalances affect your physical stress. Fatigue, lack of sleep, and dehydration are all physical stressors. Illness (viral, bacterial, or fungal) can cause short-term physical stress. Whereas diseases like diabetes, obesity, heart disease, any dis-ease can cause chronic physical stress on the body.

Chronic physical stress can also be a reaction to emotional stress such as long periods of time in a tense position—holding stress in your neck and/or shoulders or another part of your body. Postural changes along with skeletal dysfunction and muscle weakness is often a result of stress.

Physical stress starts at the nervous system, moves to the cardiovascular system, and then to the digestive system. Increased stress—pumps out more glucose, which then moves to the muscular system where muscles tighten and may lead to muscle fatigue, headaches, muscle spasms. The stress then makes its way to the immune system—acute stress will boost your immune system and fight illness. Chronic stress lowers your immune system and causes chronic inflammation. Your body's reactions to bacteria and viruses are then slower, which affects your liver and your lymphatic system, and you are more likely to get sick. Our environment and life choices have a trickle-down effect that causes physical stress to our entire body.

Physical stress is going to occur—we are humans—living human experiences. How your body systems are responding to physical stress is what's important. Are you loving, listening, and learning from the stress your body is in? Let's use exercise as an example. We know exercise is healthy for us, but an intense workout will cause physical stress to our bodies. *Does that mean I shouldn't work out?* No. Physical stress can help build your body to be stronger. Let's say you have an intense workout and thirty minutes later you are dragging and it affects you the rest of the day—this is a sign your physical stress load is too high compared to if you have a workout and thirty minutes later you have more energy—a sign, physical stress is strengthening you. Finding what your body needs and starting there and slowly progressing is how exercise can help you handle stress.

Just as many women are not aware of how much emotional stress is taking a toll on their emotional health, most women are not aware of how much physical stress is affecting their physical health. Just like emotional awareness is important. Physical awareness is important too. We often are hard on ourselves and expect more than our physical body can handle. Part of loving ourselves unconditionally and forgiving ourselves includes being nice. For years I was my biggest bully. I am now learning how to be gentle and kind to myself and others.

Knowing what your body can handle, where your body is in space, knowing where the body parts are and how they feel, how your body is moving and working, whether it is in balance or out of balance, how it feels and responds to different activities all play a part in having optimal physical health.

Remember, stress is a part of life—but you are in control of your body and you can assess how stress is affecting you and make changes. Using techniques that bring your body back to the parasympathetic mode (rest, digest, and heal) is an important daily self-care habit. Biofeedback—types of testing or technology to see how different strategies affect your physiology is a good place to start. It may be something as simple as going for a walk and asking yourself, "How is my energy level?" "Did I do too much?" "Could I have done more?" You could check your heart rate and/or blood pressure and see how deep breathing affects either or both of them. You could use a tool like checking your HRV (heart rate variability) to see how your autonomic nervous system is doing—are you in a low stressed state or high stressed state?

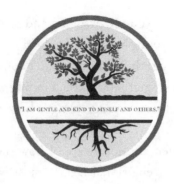

NEXT STEP

What's your next step? Research has shown deep breathing activates the vagus nerve and resets the autonomic nervous system and returns you to a parasympathetic mode, bringing hormonal balance, and decreasing stress.

Deep breathing allows you to get into the "rest, digest, and heal" stage so your gut can heal and improve your immune system by quieting it down, which is beneficial if you have allergies or autoimmune diseases.

Studies have shown when you activate the vagus nerve and spend more time in the parasympathetic stage the microbiome balances and gut infections like SIBO (Small Intestine Bacterial Overgrowth) improve in 2-3 months compared to the typical 6-8 years using drugs and diet treatment to change the gut.[7] One of the first signs you have activated your vagus nerve and in the parasympathetic mode is gurgling in the tummy because blood flow has returned to the stomach and other organs—remember the vagus nerve connects the heart, brain, lungs, liver, stomach, spleen, pancreas, and colon.

We are spiritual, emotional, and physical beings and our beliefs lead to our thoughts and affect our emotional health, which leads to how we feel. We get to choose the actions that affect our physical health and give us our results—our overall state of health and well-being. Starting your morning with deep breathing exercises will help lower stress and improve physical health.

**Go to www.shawnacale.com/book-bonus
Printable Journal Pages and Bonus Resources
to Live an Exceptional Life.**

EXERCISE: DEEP BREATHING

1. Deep Breathing Exercise: Slowly breathe in through your nose, hold the breath at the top for a comfortable amount of time. (Breath retention stimulates the vagus nerve.) Exhale through the mouth with a soft "haaa" sound like you are misting your glasses to clean them. (Sound also stimulates the vagus nerve.) Let your exhale be longer than your inhale. (The exhale is the key to strengthen vagal tone.) Continue for 2-5 minutes.

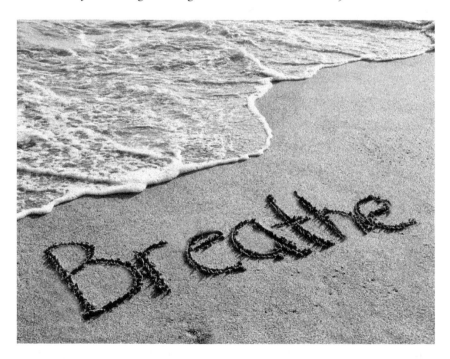

ExSEPshNL Formula: Next Step—Deep Breathing.

10

The Essentials

"Most big transformations come about from the hundreds of tiny, almost imperceptible, steps we take along the way."
~ Lori Gottlieb

Have you ever noticed as humans we celebrate the big accomplishments and pay less attention to the steps it took to get there? Even on vacations, I remember spending more time asking, "Are We There Yet?" than enjoying the actual trip. Funny thing is, many of my memories are the happenings to and from the destination than the destination itself. I believe setting goals is super important. How can you get where you want to go—if you don't know where you are going? But often we never get there because we only want the endpoint, the result, we don't want to take the daily steps to get there.

The exceptional life *is* the little steps—one belief flipped, one thought captured, one emotion released, one feeling felt, one action taken—whether it's a walk, a prayer, a time of meditation, a day of fasting, a deep breath, a good night of sleep or a big glass of water, each step leads us to where we want to be and is where the transformation occurs.

As I have shared before, our spiritual, emotional, and physical beings often have blockers we must move through to become the who that reaches the goals we have set or the results we desire. My desire was to get off the hormonal/emotional rollercoaster. What is necessary to have exceptional health? Are you ready? sh—no, it's not a secret. It's the next two letters in the ExSEPshNL Formula after the "P" and the essentials to physical health. I believe these two rings: sleep and hydration when added to the SEP Circle will bring healing to your physical body and strengthen you as you deal with all the stressors coming your way and can bring you two steps closer to getting off the hormonal/emotional rollercoaster.

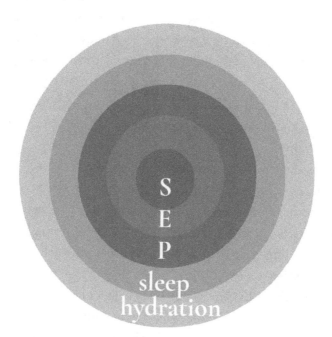

ExSEPshNL Solution: Hormonal Balance

SLEEP

"Sleep is that golden chain that ties health and our bodies together."
~ Thomas Dekker

Let's talk about sleep. Why do so many people fight it? Why do we need to sleep? Why is sleep essential for exceptional health? So many questions and as we walk through the essentials, I hope you see how sleep can give you an extra layer to strengthen YOU.

I am sure you have a cell phone, most people do these days. What happens if you don't plug in your phone? The battery dies, right? Is your phone much good if it's dead? Your body, like a cell phone battery, needs to be recharged. Sleep is necessary for our nervous and cardiovascular systems (electrical batteries) to work. Sleep allows our neurotransmitters to do their jobs and allows our neurons to shut down and repair themselves. Without sleep, toxic byproducts from the outside world, and our own normal cellular debris causes the body to malfunction. Sleep allows the brain to build neural highways that help you remember skills and habits.

Sleep also affects our hormones and helps the body's cells to increase the production of certain proteins—building blocks needed for cell growth and repair or proteins to break down damaged cells from stress and other environmental factors. We also know deep sleep—"beauty sleep" plays a huge role in how your body ages physically and mentally. Yes! Beauty sleep is a real thing.

We have what's known as our body's biological clock—this plays a part in our circadian rhythm, which is our internal clock that has a 24-hour cycle, also known as the sleep/wake cycle. I am fascinated by the organ clock that shows what time of day/night our different organs are resting and when they have their most energy. A lack of sleep plays a huge role in your physical body because of the physical stress it causes. The more physical stress to your body, the more sleep you need. Think about children growing—this is positive physical stress, yet it is still a stressor. Babies grow the most in the first 2-3 years of life and require the most sleep time—up to 16 hours a day. Most young children need up to 12 hours of sleep, and teenagers during a growth spurt can often require as much as 10-12 hours of sleep too. Everyone else needs around 8 hours of sleep, give or take an hour.

Is sleep an issue for you? Trouble falling asleep, trouble staying asleep? Sleep issues are often a result of a health blocker? Could your sleep issues be spiritual—limiting beliefs around sleep? Could a trapped emotion affect your sleep? Is your sleep a physical issue? Let's look at all three.

The spiritual side of sleep: God designed our bodies to sleep. In fact, you can find scripture after scripture where God urges us to rest in His Word. When we face difficult circumstances—when we feel like the entire world is against us—when we don't have the desire to go on. What if the most spiritual thing we can do is get a good night of sleep?

"In peace I will lie down and sleep, for you alone, O LORD, will keep me safe."

PSALM 4:8 (NLT)

What about our beliefs, how can they affect our sleep? Remember, we create most beliefs as a child. Has sleep been an issue most of your life? Could your parents have instilled the belief you were a poor sleeper? Did something traumatic happen as a child that affected your sleep? Do you have the mantra? "I just can't fall asleep." "I'm not a good sleeper." Those are limiting beliefs. Yes, I understand it may be your truth, but when that is your belief, what thoughts come up when you lie in bed? "I'll never be able to go to sleep." "I'm not tired." "If I don't go to sleep, I'm going to be grumpy tomorrow." Studies show those with more limiting beliefs (a negative attitude) have greater sleep difficulties, which also include insomnia and sleep apnea. Yet, these same people believe they need less sleep than others or live in denial their sleep issues are causing their health issues. Those that have stress-related illnesses like depression and anxiety have more sleep issues and sleep issues feed into both illnesses too.[1] It is a vicious circle that finds its way to the "normal" population. Over 68 percent of American's have sleep issues today.[2]

Do you go over all the thoughts of the day the moment you lie down—all the things that went wrong? What emotions do these types of thoughts bring up? Now how do you feel? Has this engaged your sympathetic nervous system—the *fight*-or-*flight* response? You can't fall asleep when your sympathetic nervous system is on—remember, it's like pushing the gas on the car. What action can you take to engage the brakes—your parasympathetic system—the rest and digest mode? The most simple action: deep breathing and positive affirmations. One of my favorite affirmations before bed is, "I am at peace." When you are in the parasympathetic stage, your body can rest and you can fall asleep. Your result—sleep—spiritual rest. Guess what? This can even help you change your limiting belief into an empowering belief because now you know you can fall asleep—because you did.

The emotional side of sleep: What if there is an emotion preventing you from getting a good night's sleep? The emotion most related to sleep issues—*frightened*. Now, this does not have to be an emotion you are even aware of having. You may not "feel" afraid when you are going to bed at night, but it's those trapped emotions we are not aware of that cause some of the biggest problems. We define *frightened* as afraid or anxious and is an emotion that usually occurs in childhood. The other side is peaceful. I don't know about you, but I love peace and even better a peaceful night of sleep. What if you released this emotion and embraced peace?

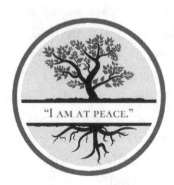

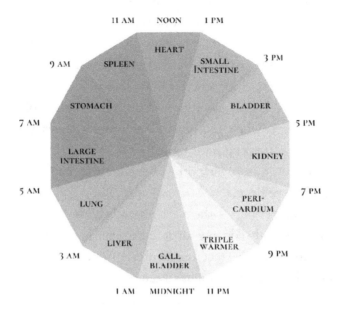

ORGAN CLOCK

Our physical health can also play a role in our ability to sleep and stay asleep. The most common period people wake up in the middle of the night is between 1:00-3:00 am. *Why is this?* Every organ has its own frequency, and it also has a time to get its major energy flow from the body to do its work and a time for rest—kind of like charging its own personal organ battery to 100%—to last until the next day.

Looking at the organ clock, this is the time the liver is finishing up the detoxing process and, if overwhelmed, could wake you up. Remember, the liver is like the "mom" its job is to keep everything clean and everything in running order. Just as many of us moms are the housekeeper, taxi driver, homework helper, cook, and the list goes on. It may seem like there is more work to be done than one can handle. *Can I get an amen?* So we wake up in the middle of the night sweating or maybe needing to go pee. Two of the ways your body helps eliminate toxins, the liver has been breaking down through the night. However, the liver has more work, and if it doesn't get time to rest, neither do you. Between 3-5 am the lungs/ respiratory system expels toxins so you may cough or get restless during this process. If you are not sleeping between 11 pm-5am, then your body cannot detoxify at its greatest capacity. This often affects those that work late-night shifts and affects hormone levels and increases the chance of obesity and diabetes. Often supporting your liver can help you get a better night's sleep.

It is essential to get a good night's sleep for overall holistic health. What's amazing is when you put into action what I have shared previously: walking, flipping limiting beliefs to empowering beliefs, emotional release, deep breathing, prayer, meditation, and fasting all have shown to improve sleep.

Bonus: Lavender one of the most researched essential oils also helps with both sleep and reducing anxiety through inhalation. It enhances vagal tone and helps balance out neurotransmitters, giving a calming effect, and allowing a good night's sleep.[3]

**Go to www.shawnacale.com/book-bonus
Printable Journal Pages and Bonus Resources
to Live an Exceptional Life.**

EXERCISE: SLEEP

1. What do you feel is your biggest blocker to sleeping 8 hours per night?

2. If you wake up at night, what time is it usually? Find the system on the Organ Clock that could use some support.

3. What is one action you could put into effect to get a better night of sleep?

HYDRATION

*"Your body requires hydration to digest your food,
to regulate your hormones, and to be able to think clearly."*
~ Mandy Ingber

Do you like water? As a child, I only liked my mom's glass of water. She would put ice and water in a big glass and then set it down. I am not sure how much of it she drank, but I know I only drank water from her glass, the water hose, and the water fountain at school until I met my husband. I am not sure why, partly because the water had little taste, I preferred something sweet like lemonade, sweet tea, or pop. Now, I drink 8 or more glasses of water each day and if you see me, there is a 99 percent chance I will have my water bottle with me. I even take jugs of my filtered water from home whenever I travel or if spending a day at someone's house. Now you may think that is excessive. I believe I spent the first half of my life dehydrated and the second half hydrated with toxic tap water. I had headaches, joint pain more days than not, and when I began drinking plenty of good filtered water, I found it kept the headaches and joint pain at bay more than anything else—even the ibuprofen I took for years. When I felt better, I didn't want to stop.

Most people have heard we can't live over 3 days without water, yet we hear about the person who never drinks water and is still alive. I lived on very little water for years, but what was it doing to my body? Yes, we can live on soft drinks, juice, energy drinks, and eat a lot to keep our fluid levels up high enough to survive. But are we healthy? Is it more food our body is needing—or it crying for water? One of my favorite books I read several years ago was *Your Bodies Many Cries for Water* by Fereydoon Batmanghelidj.[4]

Hydration is necessary for body temperature control, it lubricates your joints; gets rid of waste through urination and sweat, and keeps your bowels moving. Oh yeah, it's also necessary for your heart to beat, your blood to move, and your brain to work. Without water, your electrical system is pretty much toast. I would say hydration is pretty important!

Your body is over 70 percent water, your blood 85 percent, your brain 80 percent, your muscles are 75 percent water, and your cells that create your tissues, your organs, all that make you—90 percent water. Thirst is a sign you are dehydrated. Today 75 percent of American's are chronically dehydrated—this is the "norm" but then so is disease.

So what happens when you're dehydrated? Chronic dehydration is a disease producer. Research shows that allergies, asthma, anginal pain, chronic pain, colitis, constipation, depression, high blood pressure, high blood cholesterol, low back pain, migraine headaches, rheumatoid arthritis, obesity, could all be thirst signals.

Have you been listening to your body?

Tea, coffee, colas are all dehydrating agents because of their strong diuretic action on the kidneys. Kidneys are part of the excretory system and their job is to excrete (pee out) toxic waste products after the kidneys filter through almost 200 quarts of blood each day. Even mild dehydration has shown to cause permanent kidney damage because of the build-up of wastes and acids. Heard of kidney stones? Number one cause: You got it—dehydration. You need to urinate 1-2 quarts daily—that often looks like peeing 6-10 times a day. I know—you don't have time to pee that many times in a day—believe me, I've heard that excuse more than I can count. If you are peeing less than that or your urine is bright yellow, then you are likely *causing* physical health issues.

Dehydration can also affect mood. Did you know that UTI's (Urinary Tract Infections) often are the leading cause of confusion and disorientation? Eight glasses of water a day can keep you healthy in so many ways. Remember stress? Dehydration increases stress in your body. When you're stressed, your adrenal glands (that sit right on top of your kidneys like a hat) produce extra cortisol—the stress hormone, and under chronic stress, your adrenals can become exhausted and cause lower electrolyte levels and that's when you feel you have nothing left—**depleted.**

How about those hormones? Water flushes out toxins and helps keep hormones balanced. When we are dehydrated, we often have left-over hormones recycling through our bodies. I don't know about you, but I don't need old recycled hormones. What about fertility? For women, dehydration results in poor egg health, and less cervical mucus secretion, which is vital for the transportation of sperm to the fallopian tubes and conception.

If you had a baby, would you make sure it was well hydrated? *Why?* Because you love that baby, you want that baby to be healthy and well. Just as we make sure to take care of babies, we are responsible for our own hydration and it is a way we can love ourselves and stay healthy and well. If you haven't been loving yourself and taking care of yourself, it's okay—no judgment. Today is a new day. Forgive yourself and start new—you are full of goodness. You deserve good water to keep you healthy and well.

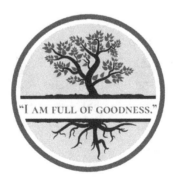

"I AM FULL OF GOODNESS."

Go to www.shawnacale.com/book-bonus
Printable Journal Pages and Bonus Resources
to Live an Exceptional Life.

EXERCISE: DRINK WATER

1. What do you feel is your biggest blocker to drinking 8 glasses of water per day?

CONSEQUENTIAL PAIN

*"Pain serves a purpose. Without it you are in danger.
What you cannot feel, you cannot take care of."*
~ Rebecca Solnit

Pain is the number #1 complaint I have heard as a physical therapist through the years. Here's the thing: Lack of sleep and dehydration play a huge role in consequential pain. I know it's not the answer you want. My patients would often roll their eyes when I would recommend 8 hours of sleep and 8 glasses of water. Or the classic, "Who has the time?" But many would then ask, "What can *you* do to decrease my pain?" That's one of the greatest problems we have in today's world. We want someone else to fix us. As I shared in my story, I was no different. Taking responsibility for my health was *not* a new concept, I taught it to my patients every day. But I realized through the process I wasn't taking care of myself in many of the essential areas and found most of our answers are in self-care habits and we don't give them the credit they deserve.

Studies link lack of sleep to increased pain, and of course pain can also cause difficulty sleeping. Pain is "natural," it's your friend telling you there is a problem. The brain will send you signals when you move something, put pressure on it, or do too much. It means stop, rest, sleep, recover. It doesn't mean take a pill and do it all like usual, this sets you up for chronic pain issues.

Believe me when I say, "I don't like pain." Nor, do I like to watch my kids or anyone else in pain. But what I have learned and watched the past 10 years without using the crutches of pain medication, over-the-counter drugs, and choosing to listen to the body and supporting the healing process has been amazing.

I have watched my daughter, Emily, go through several oral surgeries without drugs after the surgery. Ever since she was about 2 years old and had multiple ear infections and prescribed antibiotics that we forced down her throat as she vomited them back up—she cannot take or keep down drugs of any kind. Not even a Tylenol or an Ibuprofen. So you can only imagine as a mother or as the oral surgeon on what to do after surgery.

Let me just say she was a trooper—the first 24 hours was never fun—but is it ever? What we all—including the oral surgeon—learned from the experience, and what not taking meds can do to the healing process was pretty spectacular. Her healing in a week was more than most in 2 weeks. Within 48 hours she had little to no pain and most people are still on pain medication or OTC's at a week. Yes, we did things to support her body, many Epsom salt baths, essential oils on the outside and inside of her mouth, and lots of healthy smoothies.

My oldest son, Ryan, had a knee injury in a basketball game. It hurt to put weight on it, so he rested on the couch and in his bed with his leg elevated, ice, and essential oils to relieve any pain. He could have had OTC pain medication, but he chose not to. As long as he kept the weight off the leg, kept the oils and ice on it, he was fine. Within 72 hours no pain, minimal to no inflammation, and was walking without crutches or a limp. However, he had a torn meniscus and could not jump or run, so he rested the season and returned with a brace to play the next year. He wore the brace for one year and has been good for the past 7 years—no drugs, no surgery, lots of basketball. I know this is not always the case, but how often do we give our body the chance to heal?

I share these stories because our body is a wonderful healing machine when given the essentials necessary. Both of my kids slept a lot during the healing process. I kept them well hydrated. Proper hydration aids in the anti-inflammatory processes. Water puts out the cellular fire our body experiences during an injury when it has had time to heal the local area. When inflammation goes down, then the brain turns back on the vagus nerve and all is well. If the body does not have plenty of sleep and water (a chance to heal) and we slow down the process with medications or we continue to injure the area because we can't feel the pain because of the medications blocking the signals to the brain—a chronic feedback loop can continue even long after the body part is no longer injured.

I am not saying that medications are never necessary, or surgery, or both, but I am saying before you stop, block or remove—listen to your body. What does it need from you?

Even our postures and movements or lack of movements affect how our body can move and heal—the head/neck region from poor posture (forward head) often causes headaches, migraines, neck and back pain. In physical therapy school, one of the first things we learned to assess was posture. Why? Because without a healthy posture, we won't have a healthy body. Funny, how one of the first things I was told out in the field by other therapists was to just skip the posture training—it's too hard and nobody does it, anyway. So, I listened for the first few years and then decided if I was going to help people, then we needed to start at the basics. So along with sleep and hydration recommendations, I helped them learn how to improve their posture. I had an entire training program and even a cool computer program that gave them a posture number. I always knew which patients were getting plenty of sleep, water, and performing their 20 minute home exercise program that included deep breathing exercises by how well they improved. Posture changes occur when joints and vertebral discs are hydrated in the spine and the body is given time to get a good night of sleep.

Blocked pathways cause pain and discomfort and often require a multifaceted approach to facilitate healing. This is where physical therapists, chiropractors, and other holistic health practitioners can help partner with you on your healing journey. But change cannot occur if your body is not receiving the essentials it requires—that's your job. Dis-ease is the lack of energy required to allow the body to complete the healing process. Remember, we have these amazing neurotransmitters in our body and one of their jobs is to decrease pain, give them what they need and they will give you the results you desire—no pain.

> Give your body the essentials and it will heal itself.

NUTRITION

"Let food be thy medicine"
~ Hippocrates

Do you like to eat? I like to eat. I'm not sure how much I thought about what I ate nourishing my body before my journey. What I have learned is that Hippocrates once again was right—food is my medicine.

Nutrition is the next essential ring in our ExSEPshNL Formula. This ring grows or shrinks depending on what we put in our mouths. Nutrition is the science of how the body absorbs nutrients (chemical substances) from food to nourish our bodies and is essential to our health and healing. I knew nutrition was important to my health—but I never thought about the messages food was sending to my body. Yes, we all know even as a child what food is good and not so good for us, but do we understand why? Could our pain be related to what we eat? What we eat must be able to be digested by our gut. Remember, our gut is where disease and/or health begins. What we feed our microbiome affects who we are, how we feel, and what we can and cannot do.

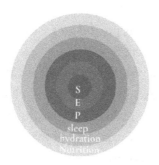

Now I shared with you my story about making several changes—like changing from tap water to filtered water and decreasing the number of processed foods in my home. But it was 40 days before my 40th birthday when I followed the *Maker's Diet*[5] and realized I was a sugar addict and an emotional eater, or maybe a better explanation was I ate to "not feel." Specifically, to "not feel" emotional or physical pain—it had nothing to do with nourishing my body. When I had a new perspective on food and how it can be a healing medicine and how many of our eating choices are drug-like, my life changed even more.

This is not a nutrition book. I will not give you a list of recipes (though I have some great ones—my Homemade Chicken soup is the best thing ever) or tell you a specific diet you should or should not follow (though I have been on many). What I want to give you are some basics I have learned over the past 10 years that may help you on your journey. Because nutrition is essential, but maybe not in the way you have thought—at least I know it wasn't for me.

Let's look at two sides of the coin: Eating and Fasting. Eating is whenever you choose to put something in your mouth that requires your body to digest. Fasting is whenever you choose to go without eating for a specific period. Did you notice the word—choose? We get to choose each day what we are going to eat. What we choose affects how we feel, how we function, and even how we make decisions throughout the day. As an adult, we get to choose what and when we eat or don't eat. Seriously, I think sometimes we forget this. We think it's time to eat and I have to eat now and the only thing around is... so it's better than nothing. *What if it's not?*

You may feel your diet is just fine, I sure did. You may think, "What I eat doesn't affect me from living out my exceptional life," and maybe that's true or maybe it's not. Maybe it's an excuse you have been telling yourself. I was full of excuses. Either way—what if you asked God for wisdom in what and when you eat? What if you followed His lead and nourished your body His way instead of the world's way?

What do we eat? I have found we eat from two categories: FOOD and CRAP. Excuse my French, but the truth of the matter is we American's live on the Standard American Diet (SAD) and it is full of crap (definition: extremely poor quality). So let's break down these two choices.

FOOD

"Good food is very often, even most often, simple food."
~ Anthony Bourdain

What is food? We define food as any chemical substance people eat or drink in order to maintain life and growth. Yes, food is chemicals—I prefer mine to be all-natural chemicals created by God from plant and animal sources to nourish my body. Remember, we are a "chemical stew" and when adding FOOD we can improve how our chemicals are working and how they build us up. I like acronyms and mnemonics—ways to remember things. FOOD is an acronym we can use to remember what to eat to nourish our bodies.

F—Fruits and vegetables. Fruit and veggies give you the vitamins, minerals, and antioxidants you need to nourish your body, and they taste great! The best part is they are REAL! One thing missing in most American diets is fiber. Fruits and vegetables are a great way to get the fiber you need. How much do we need as women? Approximately 25 grams per day. Eating a variety of fruits and vegetables as the seasons change and preferably organic will give you a step up on living a healthy lifestyle. One quick and easy way to get your daily dose of fiber—a healthy smoothie with at least 5 servings of fruit and veggies.

O—Organic protein. You want it to be free of toxic chemicals and antibiotics. Our bodies require protein to build and rebuild, we need protein to make enzymes, hormones, and other "feel good" body chemicals. Protein is also an important building block of bones, muscles, cartilage, skin, and blood. Proteins break down into amino acids that are involved in growth and development, healing and repair, normal digestion, and providing energy for your body. I learned my body feels much better when I get enough protein. How much is enough? We are all different, but the recommended amount is 46 grams of protein per day for most women. If my energy is low, I need to make sure I am getting enough protein in my diet. However, if we are not moving enough and eating too much protein for our body to use daily, we may find it affects our blood sugar levels. Protein breaks down into glucose and we either burn or store it, but most women today are sedentary, which means we are not moving much and it's more likely being stored (aka fat). A quick and easy way to get your daily dose of protein in a day—3 egg omelet with veggies and cheese for one meal and 3 oz of any meat with a side of veggies for another meal.

O—Omega-3 fatty acids, are the good fats that your body can use for energy, growth, and repair. Most of us get plenty of omegas 6's and 9's, but 3's not so much. An excellent source of healthy fats is salmon, avocados, flax seeds, chia seeds, and nuts. Remember Omega-3's turn off the inflammatory response. So how much do you need? If you do not have acute or chronic inflammation, then 250-500 mg per day is enough. If you are dealing with acute or chronic inflammation, then 500-2,000 mg per day. Remember, if you have a disease of any kind—it's because of chronic inflammation. Unless you are having salmon, several times a week it is very difficult to get enough Omega 3's from your diet and why most people in America need to supplement. A quick and easy way to get your daily dose of Omega-3's—Choose a Fatty Fish like Salmon a few times a week for your meat, add avocado, nuts and sprinkle chia seeds and flax seeds in smoothies and on salads.

I had a blood test a few years ago that not only gave me my CRP level which was 1.5 mg/L (optimal for women is less than 1.0 mg/L) meaning that I had some inflammation—remember that greater than 10.0 mg/L considered the disease level. However, my report also showed my Omega 3 index which was 3.6 (optimal >8) Which means my Omega-3 Fatty Acids were low and unable to turn off my inflammatory response. I needed to add Omega 3's to my diet, or I was on the road leading me to chronic inflammation and chronic disease. I choose to take the Omega-3 road.

D—Drink water. I know we already discussed hydration, but water is very important for your body to get the nutrients it needs. Yes, water is the most common nutrient in our body. Many chemical processes take place in water and when we choose real food from these categories along with enough water, we build a strong healthy foundation.

FOOD is real and gives our body what it needs. Easy enough, right? So why do we make eating healthy so difficult? For most of us, we have a habit of eating products that do not build our body up but break our body down. We may have addictions or just prefer certain things that don't nourish our bodies. Changing a lifetime of eating habits takes time and patience. Change is not always easy, but it is possible. Using the FOOD acronym as a guide, start adding in FOOD—Fruits and vegetables, Organic protein, Omega-3 Fats, and Drink more water daily to nourish your body.

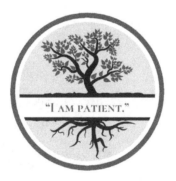

"I AM PATIENT."

Go to www.shawnacale.com/book-bonus
Printable Journal Pages and Bonus Resources
to Live an Exceptional Life.

EXERCISE: NOURISH YOUR BODY

1. What do you feel is your biggest blocker to eating FOOD to nourish your body daily?

2. How can you make eating FOOD simple today?

SIMPLE MEAL IDEAS

Monday—Wednesday—Friday:

Smoothie for breakfast, Green Leafy Salad with 3 oz of organic protein for lunch, and fatty fish and veggies for dinner.

Tuesday—Thursday—Saturday:

Omelet for breakfast, Smoothie for lunch, and 3 oz of organic protein with veggies for dinner.

Sunday:

Enjoy a casserole, soup, or chili full of veggies, organic protein, and Omega-3's. Dessert of fruit and nuts.

CRAP

"Eat like crap. Feel like crap. Look like crap."
~ Unknown

How did I not know for so many years the CRAP I was eating was making me feel the way I felt? I mean, don't get me wrong. When I eat sweets, processed foods, chips, candy—at that moment—I feel great. All is well with the world. Sometimes I don't feel so well a few hours later, but it's the next day when I have forgotten what I even ate the day before and on to finding something else to eat to make me feel better. It's at that moment that yesterday's choices really affect me. My day after is often a headache, sometimes a bellyache, but mostly it's just a mood thing. I'm just really ticked off and I don't even know why—except now I do. Because I used to eat CRAP every day and felt like crap every day, I didn't realize it was what I ate that made me feel bad until... it's amazing we don't know how good we can feel until we feel good.

Though many think of CRAP as food, let's be clear it consists of synthetic (man-made) chemicals that break down our body, not build it up. Just like FOOD, I have an acronym for what we don't want to put in our body on a daily basis.

C—Carbonated drinks-aka soda that includes caffeine, sugar, and other substances that have a negative effect on our body. Often, the elimination of soda can be a significant step towards living a lifestyle of wellness. An average 20 oz bottle of pop has about 16 teaspoons of sugar inside of it. For the longest time, the major brands have tried to deny the fact that science shows a clear link between sugar consumption and obesity. The first soda drinks were 'born' in the 1850s in the local drugstore to cure physical ailments. Many fountain drinks were concoctions or extracts or flavored effervesced drugs. Cocaine and caffeine were among the most popular drugs of choice, and they used the combination as a headache treatment. Patients would then suffer rebound headaches and would return for more drinks to treat their pain. Some things haven't changed except instead of cocaine in the drink we have high amounts of sugar or we just grab an OTC along with our soda to relieve the headache and have the same rebound headaches that have us grabbing the bottle or drink, day after day. This type of addiction often leads us to prescription medications, alcohol, and even illegal drugs.

R—Refined sugars, which have no nutritional value. The refinement process takes out anything nutritional from the plant and uses chemicals for the processing. Now you may think, how is this different from sugars in fruit? Fruit contains vitamins, minerals, and fiber. The presence of fiber also minimizes the effect of glucose on our bloodstream by slowing down the rate of digestion. As a result, we will experience a much slower rise in insulin by consuming a banana versus eating a piece of candy or chocolate cake. Studies have shown refined sugar is a drug. Brain scans have confirmed, refined sugar affects the brain in ways similar to certain drugs. The Journal of *Neuroscience and Biobehavioral Reviews* found refined sugar meets the criteria as *a substance of abuse* and may be addictive to those that eat it.[6] Animal studies show refined sugar to be more addictive than cocaine, and refined sugar is the most consumed addictive substance around the world. We can find it in white bread, cookies, pastries, candy, breakfast cereals, fruit drinks, soda, and many other processed foods. Most sugar addictions start in childhood and are the "norm" for most children today who are not even aware of the destruction it is causing to their health or their future. Cutting back on refined sugar, or sugars will also give your pancreas a break from pumping out insulin. Bye, bye insulin resistance!

A—Artificial sweeteners and colors are not "real," hence the term "artificial." Many people are allergic to artificial sweeteners and colors. Especially red dye. *Many children have a red dye specific allergy.* Lesser known are the effects of aspartame. They have reported it to be the culprit behind many headache sufferers. Sometimes it's caused vision impairment and neurological symptoms. Artificial sweeteners are worse than refined sugar, *that's right, you heard me.* **WORSE!** Our body can process sugar because it has been in our diet since day one. But artificial sweeteners taste just as sweet without using sugar. *It's not natural, and it's not REAL!* As far as colors go, they are toxic chemicals. When you consume artificial colors, you are consuming dye. All that colorful candy that is so fun to eat has dyes in it. Anyone want some blue#2—Oh yeah, it's also linked to brain tumors? I didn't think so. If you want your food or drink to be a certain color, you can find a version where the color is derived from vegetables. Better yet, if you want a rainbow of colors to eat, just look at all the fruits and vegetables available to you.

P—Processed food. Pretty much all fast food is highly processed. Cutting back your fast food intake can help improve health, there is nothing beneficial to eating processed food. Some argue you can get protein from a burger or chicken fingers, but what else are you getting with it? Is your body even taking it in as nourishment or seeing it as another toxin and fighting it with the inflammatory response? Fast food is not the only culprit, much of the boxed foods, white pasta, potato chips, processed cheeses, cereals, and refined flours are just as toxic to our body. Remember the White Flour Tortilla story? Me and refined sugar mixed with refined white flour is a chemistry experiment gone bad—picture the red and blue beakers poured into the flask and an explosion occurs—that's me and it's not a good thing.

CRAP is *"fake food"* our body cannot process efficiently and causes physical stress, which then affects our body from absorbing nutrients from our "real" food. Remember, "normal" American adults are malnourished and overweight from poor diets. Sadly, the number of children that are now overweight and obese is rising, and 1 in 5 children fall in this category. Have you caught onto the pattern yet? CRAP: Carbonated drinks, Refined sugar, Artificial sweeteners & colors, and Processed foods are not real. They were all created by scientists, and because of the chemical process they undergo, the body cannot digest them properly. We have to stop the CRAP so our body does not have to cleanse itself of harmful toxins.

"I have the right to do anything," you say—but not everything is beneficial. "I have the right to do anything"—but I will not be mastered by anything.
1 CORINTHIANS 6:12 (NIV)

Eating foods in their most natural state allows the body to take in nutrients and fuel from the food nature intended. CRAP is also highly addictive. If you have been eating processed food for an extended period, your taste buds have adjusted to accept the chemical form. Switching over to natural food might at first taste strange, but your taste buds will adjust and you will find natural food is very flavorful. Even all the green stuff. So next time you are ready to eat, remember to eat less CRAP and eat more FOOD. You will then have less STRESS and more ENERGY.

Go to www.shawnacale.com/book-bonus
Printable Journal Pages and Bonus Resources
to Live an Exceptional Life.

ACTION: BYE BYE CRAP

1. Choose FOOD—not CRAP the next time you go grocery shopping. Even better, find a local Farmer's Market so you don't have as many temptations to choose from.

2. What is one step you can take today to decrease the amount of CRAP you eat?

FASTING

"The best of all medicines are resting and fasting."
~ Benjamin Franklin

Fasting- does the word make you cringe? Does it feel impossible? That's where I was for years. I mean, I would get "Hangry" if I went over 2-3 waking hours without eating. How could I live without putting something in my mouth for days?

Now we often think the only way we can nourish our body is by eating, even if that means choosing to eat that which is not good for us. But did you know that fasting may be just as essential to our health as eating, if not more so? I know this may be a foreign concept to you—it was for me, but follow me down this road and see if this could be beneficial to you.

First, let's start with the thought of balance. If we have 24 hours in a day and eat within a 12-hour period and fast for a 12-hour period—wouldn't that be balanced? Did you know until the 1980s that 12-hour fasting was the "norm" in America? You would eat dinner around 6 pm and eat breakfast around 6-7 am. No snacking in between. *What is breakfast?* It just means you are breaking the fast. It wasn't until the 80s that snacking became popular and fasting went to the wayside. And breakfast got a whole new meaning. People are up until 11 pm or later snacking and then get up tired and starving in the morning because of the sugar rush all night. Then they grab a bowl of processed cereal full of sugar to get a little energy at 7 am to break that very short fast and then need a snack by 9 or 10 am. *Or was that just me?*

I have found breakfast to be the most important meal—but not the way commercials tell us, but because after you fast your cells are ready and prepared to be nourished, um I wouldn't say the "normal" breakfast—donuts, bagels, cereal is very nourishing. And to be clear, breakfast doesn't have to happen before noon. Guess when obesity and diabetes rose? Yep! The 80s. The music was outstanding—our food choices were not so good. We were told to stop eating fat and eat every 2-3 hours to keep up our metabolism. I think we can agree that was a big mistake! Healthy fats (remember those Omega 3's) keep down the inflammation, keep us feeling full, and keep our hormones and happy neurotransmitters balanced. Instead, we replaced the fat with sugar, lots of sugar.

So what happens when we are not eating—aka "fasting?" Fasting stimulates the body's ability to repair, it has a metabolism-boosting effect and increases growth hormone levels, which is important for our brain and other organs. Now the biggest myth about fasting I believed for way too long was it would cause nutrient deficiencies. Did you know many nutrients are not absorbed at the time we eat them? Our body is amazing, so it stores it in our liver, our muscles, and our fat cells and the only way we can get to them for nourishment is when we are fasting. That's right! Our body was made to nourish us when we are not eating! When we eat all day and even all night, our body doesn't have the time to digest what we already have and our body is storing and waiting for us to fast.

Fasting boosts the immune system, decreases inflammation, and helps decrease chronic pain too. It stimulates the clean-up and recycling of damaged cells, improves DNA repair, improves insulin sensitivity, and protects you from several diseases. Fasting slows down aging and increases overall fat burning. Fasting increases energy levels, helps you to focus, think more clearly, and improves mood. From the girl who got "Hangry" if she didn't eat every 2-3 hours, this was a tremendous surprise. Now it took time to work up to not eating every few hours, but now I can go 16-18 hours with no problem and found that fasting 36 hours once a week made the biggest shift in my blood sugar levels. Five years of different (healthy eating) diets that focused on blood sugar control kept me insulin resistant (one step from pre-diabetes and two steps from diabetes). When I began fasting, my morning blood glucose levels decreased from as high as 120 to the low 90s. Fasting is also how I lost 30 pounds in 6 months while traveling half of that time in our RV and enjoyed the occasional sweet treat. I went without sugar for 9 months doing the Keto Diet a few years ago and lost less than 5 pounds and woke up every morning with a blood glucose level above 100. My body never had time to rest—I was too busy eating all the healthy foods and getting enough fat to get into ketosis, which means fat burning. I would spend all my time trying to pick out all the right foods to get into ketosis and found later that after 12-16 hours of fasting I could get to the same level that it would take me 3-4 days of eating Keto style. It only took 36 hours of fasting to get me to the same level of ketosis as 3-4 weeks of eating Keto. Sometimes we make things more difficult than they have to be. Now I am not saying Keto is not an option, nor any of the other diets I or possibly you have done, but I am saying it may not be the food we are eating as much as the fact we never stop eating.

What about all the "normal" diseases we see today—arthritis, asthma, allergies, cancer, diabetes, heart disease, obesity, Alzheimer's, and other neurological diseases? I have found in my research fasting slows down these processes and often even prevents overall chronic disease when part of a healthy lifestyle. A scientific review in the *Journal of Obesity* found that fasting may be more healthful than other dieting strategies and allow the body to become more efficient in utilizing fat for energy over glucose.[7] I agree.

How does fasting work? It allows your body to rest, renew, and regenerate because it's not needing to spend all its time digesting food.

It also allows genes to turn on so it can repair cells and even increase proteins to help decrease depression, anxiety, and dementia. One of the most amazing aspects of fasting is that it allows *autophagy* to occur, which is like the body's garbage-disposal system inside of cells and gets rid of damaged molecules, and uses them to tap into the nutrients we need. Damaged cells have been linked to diseases such as Alzheimers, Parkinson's, and cancer. Fasting has also been shown to reduce cancers and even maximize the positive effects of chemotherapy. Tumor cells show less growth and normal cells thrive and are even protected during fasting.[8] Women that fasted 13 hours a day (8 of that while sleeping) had fewer recurrences of breast cancer.[9] Think about that, stop eating at 6 pm and have your first meal at 7 am and your overall health improves and may even prevent cancer.

How many women do you know trying to lose weight? Are you? One question I hear so often is, "What should I eat to lose weight?" I was guilty of asking this same question for years. But let's think about that question for just a minute. What happens when we eat in the first place? When looking at how the law of mathematics works, if you add food to your body, you will also add weight. This is a good thing, so we don't waste away. But we in America are not wasting away—we are malnourished but that is two different things. We are in one of two states at all times, fed or fasted. Either we are taking in food—eating and storing calories and our gut is working at digesting or we are fasting and our digestive system is at rest and we are burning stored calories. When do you think you lose weight? If you said while fasting, you were correct. Most of us spend most of our time in the fed state and very little time in the fasted/rest state. So what happens? We gain weight! Do you know how long it takes your body to digest a meal? As little as 16 hours and up to 24 hours if you're hydrated and getting enough fiber, and your gut works as it should, for many that is not the case, and food can linger for days. A healthy weight occurs when we are in a caloric balanced state—that cannot happen if we are eating non stop, even if it is good healthy food. I did not understand this concept until I began studying how fasting worked.

So why don't we think about fasting anymore? I believe in the past people didn't think about fasting; it was just part of their lifestyle—they listened to their body. Today, it's just not part of our "normal" culture, so we have to be taught and begin living it again. Just as walking, deep breathing, prayer, and meditation are important and free—fasting costs nothing and nobody is making money selling it—so it's not on every commercial or billboard.

This brings us to the next excuse that I hear, "I can't afford to get healthy." Being healthy does not cost more—disease costs more. How much would your grocery bill decrease if you weren't buying snacks? What if you ate 1-2 meals per day so you could spend more on organic food and/or your kids could eat 3 meals of real food? Now I am not talking about starving here. I'm just saying we eat way more than we need. *How many calories do you need a day to survive?* Do you know? A "normal" American eats 3600 or more calories per day. A sedentary woman requires ~1600 calories a day to stay at her current weight and up to 2400 calories for a woman that is active or supporting a baby or breastfeeding. If you want to lose weight—your body must eat from your current food storage—aka fat. To do that, you must give your body the ability to do it. I find it much easier to eat two 600-800 calorie meals a day than three 300-600 calorie meals a day, but everyone is different.

Now there are all kinds of "fasts" out there—there is what people call intermittent fasting, the fasting-mimicking diet, water fasts, juice fasts, etc. I believe we can keep it simple by eating FOOD in a window of 8-12 hours and fasting while only drinking water for the rest of the time. If you would like to find out more about fasting, there is a ton of information available. My favorite two books—*Fast Your Way to Health* by Lee Bueno[10] is a book that sat on my bookshelf for over 5 years before I passed it one day and God said, "Now!" I read it and was so intrigued. I knew I had fasted a few times in my life and thinking back I had excellent results. This book was from a spiritual perspective and uses prayer and fasting together. It was this book that led me to fast the same week I realized *conditional* love was a limiting belief blocking me from moving forward on my exceptional health journey. Would I have been as open to this concept if I had not been praying, meditating, and fasting at the time? I'm not sure. I do believe they were part of the emotional healing process.

The second book I read was from a scientific perspective, *The Complete Guide to Fasting* by Jason Fung.[11] Much like my introduction to essential oils, first, from a biblical and then from a scientific perspective, I could see how fasting could be beneficial to me and others. As I have experimented, I have seen wonderful results. Many people ask if they should take supplements or medications while fasting. Most people can fast 12 hours—remember this was "normal" forty years ago and continue with their supplement or medication schedule after they break the fast. If you are going to do longer fasts and you're on medications, it is always best to discuss this with your doctor. I recommend you do your own research, remember you are the CEO of your own health and need to make your own decisions. I supplement during my eating time window and choose not to take anything by mouth except water during my fasting periods. However, I use essential oils and/or Epsom salt baths during fasting to support my body as needed.

Go to www.shawnacale.com/book-bonus
Printable Journal Pages and Bonus Resources
to Live an Exceptional Life.

ACTION: EATING AND FASTING

1. **Beginner**: Start by eating 3 meals a day in a 12-hour period with no snacks and see how you feel.

2. **Advanced:** Increase your fasting window and decrease your eating window until you reach the results and goals you are working towards.

NEXT STEP

I know I just took you down a hard road, at least it has been for me. The "normal" road seems so "normal" right? How do we say "No," to what we have grown up eating, enjoying, finding pleasure in? We look at the exceptional road and think—is this what I really want? Do I want to be deprived of all the "sweets" of life? I understand. Here's what I have found. My hormonal/emotional rollercoaster and pain improved when the essentials became a part of my daily routine. When I eat real food, I stop craving all the junk. I do not feel like I am missing out or being deprived. *I feel good.* But it doesn't take much of the refined sugar and flour to get me back on the addiction train and screaming for more. I pay the consequences and think I'll say no next time, but then it happens again. I am still a work in progress and what I've learned is to stop beating myself up, because that doesn't help the problem—it causes the problem—stress.

The solution I have found is when I follow the ExSEPshNL Formula and take each day, each choice one step at a time, I make choices that feel good based on how I can best love myself at that moment. Do I mess up? You bet! Then I ask myself and often those around me to forgive me. I commit to doing better the next time, and I learn. What I have learned on this journey is patience. Patience with me. Patience with others. Change takes time, flipping beliefs, releasing emotions and the ability to stop and listen to my body on what it needs is a process. But it's not impossible. Because I believe anything is possible. I am worthy of being healthy spiritually, emotionally, and physically. I want you to know it's possible for you too. You can have happy hormonal balance. You are worthy of an exceptional life.

The three essentials: sleep, hydration, and nutrition build us up and keep us strong. We are in control of how much we sleep, how much water we drink, and what and when we eat. These are the foundation for happy, healthy hormones. I believe sleeping for 8 hours, drinking 8 glasses of water, eating real food a portion of our day (for me in an 8-hour window), and fasting the rest is essential to have exceptional health. It's even easy to remember 8-8-8, and each one is part of my 8 Steps to Happy Hormonal Balance. When we do these simple actions, our results are astounding. It's not always going to be perfect, we will have sleepless nights, we will have days we drink less water, we will have days we feast more than we fast, but taking the steps towards the right direction is always better than staying on the "normal" road. If you want less stress, to feel better, and more energy, these essentials are your next step.

 Go to www.shawnacale.com/book-bonus Printable Journal Pages and Bonus Resources to Live an Exceptional Life.

EXERCISE: 8 STEPS TO HAPPY HORMONAL BALANCE

1. Ex: Walk 30 minutes per day.

2. S: Love yourself unconditionally.

3. E: Forgive yourself daily.

4. P: Deep breathing exercises daily to tell your body it is safe.

5. s: Sleep 8 hours each night.

6. h: Drink 8 glasses of water each day.

7. N: Eat more hormone balancing FOOD.

8. N: Eat less hormone-disrupting CRAP.

ExSEPshNL Formula: Next Step—Sleep, Hydrate and Nourish.

11

⥤⥂

Your Life Is Now

"Don't wait for everything to be perfect
before you decide to enjoy your life."
~ Joyce Meyer

I am happy you and I have been able to walk and talk together through the ExSEPshNL Formula. We have now reached the last letter, which is "L" for LIFE. God even gave me a mnemonic for it too. L is for Living, I is for Investing, F is for Finances and E is for Energy. Again, as we grow in each of these areas, we are adding more and more rings to our being and strengthening who we are.

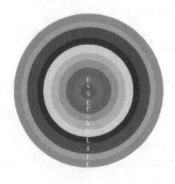

226

In living a healthy lifestyle, setting and reaching health goals, I have found that we—and I say we because I include me—use life as an excuse. "I don't have time to do it, my *life* is too busy." "When *life* slows down I'll get to it." "*Life* is just too crazy to think about it right now." "Maybe in another lifetime." Our life is right now—today. Yesterday is gone and tomorrow may never come, but what we did or didn't do yesterday affects us today and what we do today affects who we are tomorrow. I always found these thoughts a little confusing. Do I live today like there is no tomorrow? If so, why would my health even matter, do I even matter?

What if today was your last day of life on this earth—what would you do? I think we often joke about all the junk food we would eat, all the places we would want to see, but, having watched those both young and old die before me, it all comes down to spending time with those we love—our family and friends. We often hear regrets from both sides of not letting them know how much we love and appreciate them. So what if that is what we did every day? We started our day loving others and loving ourselves enough to stay as healthy as we can to have as many "today's" as possible with those we love. That for me is what I learned in January 2010 while lying in an ambulance and then in a hospital bed wondering about my tomorrow. I didn't dream about ice cream or potato chips or seeing the Eiffel Tower. I thought about my family—my mom, my husband, each of my children in my house praying for me—for my health. I didn't want to just survive and continue the life I had been living. I wanted more. I wanted to live my life on purpose for a purpose.

Is LIFE really getting in your way of being healthy?

On my journey, I have learned it's not life that blocks us from living fully—sure circumstances happen, things out of our control occur, but life-—it's the time we have between birth and death, it's our capacity for growth, reproduction, functional activity, and continual change preceding death.

If it feels like LIFE gets in the way of you living, then it's time to create the LIFE you desire. In this chapter of LIFE we are going to continue our journey down the exceptional road and at the end create our Exceptional Road Map with our exceptional morning, day, and evening routine.

We started this journey exiting off the normal road and choosing the exceptional road, the one that leads to an abundant life. One where we live by example and grow into the person God created us to be. We looked inside to our spiritual being, to our why—our beliefs. Flipping limiting beliefs like conditional love to unconditional love with affirmations like "I begin this day with (unconditional) love in my heart."

We then began walking towards our emotional being, the one that connects us to that which lies outside of us. It's how we grow our emotional intelligence to handle the stressors that come into our life by responding with love and grace instead of reacting out of fear and blame. We began releasing trapped emotions, heart walls blocking us from feeling the joy and happiness we desire. We have forgiven others, and we have forgiven ourselves with affirmations like "I forgive myself and others.." As we continued to walk through loving and forgiving our physical beings, we learned more about our amazing body and what we can do to take care of it daily. We learned self-care isn't selfish, but our God-given responsibility while we live in this body on earth. We talked about walking, deep breathing, sleeping, hydrating, and eating nourishing food. No longer do we need to use the excuse that life is getting in the way of our goals, our health, or even our dreams. Yes, we may need to plan, prepare, and to put into action that which we have learned through the ExSEPshNL Formula, but we now see the road available for every one of us. Now, as we look through this experience, we can move forward to the four areas of LIFE. Living out our purpose, investing in others, finances, and energy to do the things we love.

ExSEPshNL Solution: More Energy

LIVING

"Doing what you love each day is what makes life worth living."
~ Unknown

I believe God created each of us for a purpose. I also believe we each have our own "callings" throughout life that allows us to live out our purpose on purpose. It's what motivates us to get up in the morning, it guides us on making our life decisions, it's the "road" we travel. But, I think so often we think "living" is just getting through another day, we get up out of obligation to the world with often no vision, no goal, no direction and we live a life without purpose or searching for our purpose as we follow the world down the "normal" road, not knowing where it is taking us.

Are you living out your life on purpose for a purpose?
Do you feel fulfilled in what you are doing?
Do you get up in the morning filled with joy and excitement?

I don't know about you, but I think I've made living life harder than it has to be. For so long I searched for my purpose—thinking I would find it in the perfect "job" meant just for me. Is my purpose "working" as a physical therapist? Is my purpose being a stay-at-home mom? Is my purpose homeschooling, running a business, being a coach? Am I missing it altogether? What if I was asking the wrong questions? What if my purpose is to love—love God, love others, and love myself every day?

When I look at my purpose from that perspective, it opens up living my life in a whole new way. Every day I can ask myself, "How can I love today?" It allows me to use my gifts and fulfill my callings. I believe I was called to be a physical therapist—the years I helped people with that calling was not only a blessing to me, but to so many others—I could love them with patience and kindness. It also brought people into my life I could show God's, unconditional love. When I had my first son—Ryan, I was called into motherhood. Every day I have been able to live out my purpose by loving him as only a mother can love. Then the Lord blessed my womb with more and I could love even more children, both those in heaven and on earth. I have been able to love my little girl, Emily, and pray for her and help lead her down a road that looks different from the road I traveled. I can love my son Bryce as a wiser and more experienced mom. When I was called to homeschool it gave me the opportunity to love each of my children throughout the day by teaching them, guiding them, investing in their future, being their safe place. When I was called to work from home and started my own health and wellness business, I could love others by sharing exceptional wellness products and services that could benefit them and their families. When I was called to write this book, it was so I could love you with words, share my experiences, my knowledge, and my gifts.

There is no shortage of callings in this world that allows us to live out our purpose. There is no limit on the number of people whom we can help inspire or support. There is no cap on the number of passions we can pursue.

Maybe you are living out your life purpose every day and have been totally aware of it. Or maybe, like me, you have been searching to find your life purpose and though it is right there, it's as if you are blind and deaf to what it is. I believe my heart wall was blocking me from seeing my purpose for so long. I could feel it deep down, but it felt so far out of reach. I once read in an article that your purpose is often like a "compass or lighthouse that provides an overarching aim and direction in day-to-day lives." [1] As I shared before, the word exceptional was like a beacon or a lighthouse to direct me on my path—leading me to see my purpose. It wasn't until I was writing this book—right here, right now, that I realized my full purpose—exceptional love.

It's funny how we can go full circle, and I am reminded of how I began this book with a quote from Helen Keller. I remember one day thinking about how wise Helen became without the use of her eyes or her ears. I remember watching the movie about her when I was young and read her autobiography just a few years ago. [2]

THE STORY OF MY LIFE

BY HELEN KELLER

PART 1—CHAPTER 6

I remember the morning that I first asked the meaning of the word, "love." This was before I knew many words. I had found a few early violets in the garden and brought them to my teacher. She tried to kiss me: but at that time I did not like to have any one kiss me except my mother. Miss Sullivan put her arm gently round me and spelled into my hand, "I love Helen."

"What is love?" I asked.

She drew me closer to her and said, "It is here," pointing to my heart, whose beats I was conscious of for the first time. Her words puzzled me very much because I did not then understand anything unless I touched it.

I smelt the violets in her hand and asked, half in words, half in signs, a question which meant, "Is love the sweetness of flowers?"

"No," said my teacher.

Again I thought. The warm sun was shining on us.

"Is this not love?" I asked, pointing in the direction from which the heat came. "Is this not love?"

It seemed to me that there could be nothing more beautiful than the sun, whose warmth makes all things grow. But Miss Sullivan shook her head, and I was greatly puzzled and disappointed. I thought it strange that my teacher could not show me love.

A day or two afterward I was stringing beads of different sizes in symmetrical groups–two large beads, three small ones, and so on. I had made many mistakes, and Miss Sullivan had pointed them out again and again with gentle patience. Finally I noticed a very obvious error in the sequence and for an instant I concentrated my attention on the lesson and tried to think how I should have arranged the beads. Miss Sullivan touched my forehead and spelled with decided emphasis, "Think."

In a flash I knew that the word was the name of the process that was going on in my head. This was my first conscious perception of an abstract idea.

For a long time I was still–I was not thinking of the beads in my lap, but trying to find a meaning for "love" in the light of this new idea. The sun had been under a cloud all day, and there had been brief showers; but suddenly the sun broke forth in all its southern splendour.

Again, I asked my teacher, "Is this not love?"

"Love is something like the clouds that were in the sky before the sun came out," she replied. Then in simpler words than these, which at that time I could not have understood, she explained: "You cannot touch the clouds, you know; but you feel the rain and know how glad the flowers and the thirsty earth are to have it after a hot day. You cannot touch love either; but you feel the sweetness that it pours into everything. Without love you would not be happy or want to play."

The beautiful truth burst upon my mind–I felt that there were invisible lines stretched between my spirit and the spirits of others.[2]

Helen, a woman by the world's standards, had no purpose. Her life was full of obstacles, yet she did not let that stop her from living life and making a difference in this world. It is said Helen was able to learn, love, and prosper until her death of natural causes at 87. She was a true role model and lived an exceptional life.

For many of us we have been so exhausted from life—feeling like the world's problems are too big, or we are too small and just don't have the energy to live out what matters the most to us, we can't see our purpose, our gifts or our callings.

A few things to think about in living life: What drives you, energizes you, what makes you want to get out of bed in the morning? If you don't have the answer, spend some time in prayer, meditation, and fasting. Like Helen and myself, I believe you will find the answers.

Writing this book, fulfilling the calling the Lord gave me in 2011, and walking down this road of faith step by step has allowed me to live out my purpose—loving you through words of hope and healing.

Are you doing what you love each day for a living? Are you choosing to do something you don't love to make money? Are you being held back from doing what you love because you don't believe enough in yourself to fulfill that which you have been called to do?

God answered my prayers at the end of July 2011 when He gave me the opportunity to build a business from home that would allow me to do what I love to do—help people with their health and also be a stay-at-home mom. I now get to do what I love to do every day—love on my family and love on people—specifically women looking to improve their health, and I am grateful that this road has shown me that "I am enough." I am living an exceptional life.

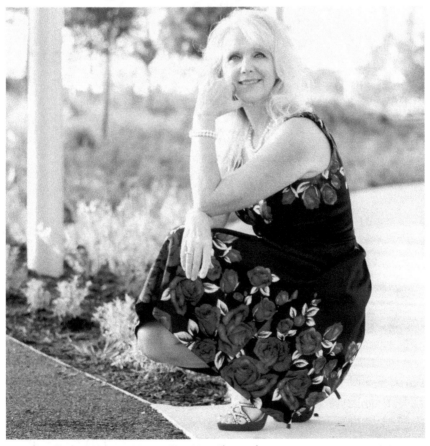

Sonja Marie Photography

Go to www.shawnacale.com/book-bonus
Printable Journal Pages and Bonus Resources
to Live an Exceptional Life.

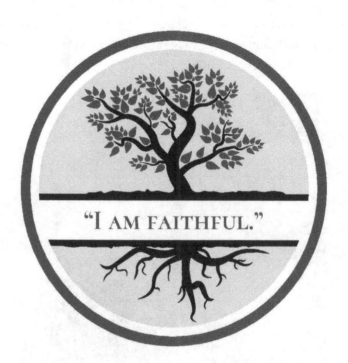

EXERCISE: LIVING A LIFE YOU DESIRE

1. What you are most passionate about, love, and naturally do best? Often as adults, we forget to dream. Have faith that your dreams are possible. If what you do for a living requires money to live on, know people every day do what they love, and make money to support their family. If they can do it, so can you! Take one step towards the life you desire today.

INVESTING

"Transformation in the world happens when people are healed
and start investing in other people."
~ Michael W. Smith

When the Lord gave me Investing for "I" in LIFE, I wasn't sure what He meant. Did I need to invest more of our money somewhere? While praying He reminded me of what my good friend Karen had told me a few years before—our time raising our children and homeschooling them was an investment into their future, our future. We were investing in our children. It changed my perspective on not only my purpose in life and my calling at that moment in time, but the purpose behind it—love.

Investing is to provide or entrust someone or something with a gift, quality, or attribute with a greater return than the original. Did you know *you* are an investment? God entrusted you with life, your gifts, and talents for a purpose. The word "investment" originally comes from the idea of being clothed. Specifically, being clothed in the official robes for a particular role. God has big plans for you. You get to decide if you are going to store up His investment—or pour it out through your life into others for a greater return.

Investing our time, our money, our gifts, our service is part of living an exceptional life. We feel good when we serve because we get what researchers call "helpers high," or a distinct physical sensation associated with helping. Want to guess what it increases? Oxytocin our "love hormone." Studies have shown people feel stronger, more energetic after helping others; many reported feeling calmer, less depressed, with increased feelings of self-worth and happiness.[3]

Remember when I shared what SEP means: "to touch, bind, join," in plain English defined as "to serve." When our spiritual, emotional, and physical hearts are connected through love and we have holistic health we serve.

Years ago I was told we find joy in serving and we can use the letters

J-O-Y to remind us who to serve. J- Jesus, O- Others, and Y-Yourself. I have taught this forever to my children and others, but in 2019 I felt like I was still looking for joy in my own life. I even hired a coach who promised to help me find joy in the journey. I learned so much through the coaching process and each step helped lead me to what I was missing—that serving is loving and I had a cup of JO, not a cup of JOY. I was loving Jesus, and I was loving Others, but my cup was not overflowing, because I was not loving myself. When I understood, JOY included me loving myself unconditionally, and investing in myself daily—releasing my heart-wall, letting go of perfection, and listening to the little girl inside. I felt the joy in the journey.

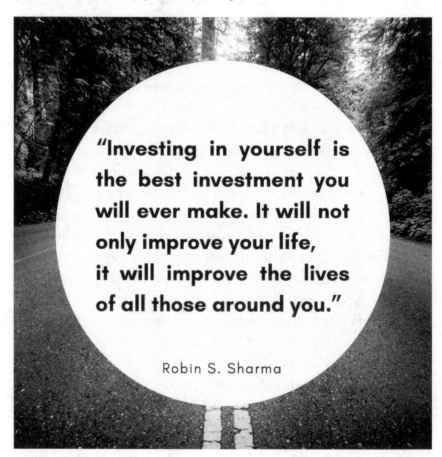

"Investing in yourself is the best investment you will ever make. It will not only improve your life, it will improve the lives of all those around you."

Robin S. Sharma

Go to www.shawnacale.com/book-bonus
Printable Journal Pages and Bonus Resources
to Live an Exceptional Life.

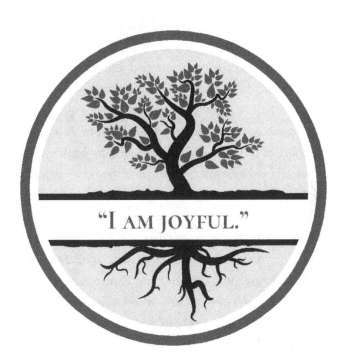

"I AM JOYFUL."

EXERCISE: INVEST IN YOUR FUTURE

1. Where are you currently investing your time, money, and energy?

2. Are you using your gifts to serve others?

3. Are you loving yourself and investing in self-care daily?

4. Do you have joy or is something missing?

FINANCES

"Financial health is restored in two ways –first
by doing the inner work of changing how you think and feel about money
and then by doing the outer work of practical money management."
~ Marianne Williamson

Financial health plays a huge part in our overall well-being. According to the American Psychological Association, money is the top cause of stress in the United States and in 2015 over 72 percent of American's reported being stressed about money.[4] Money is one of the first excuses "normal" Americans uses when it comes to eating healthy.

There is a direct correlation between health and wealth. Studies have shown a positive correlation between good health and higher income levels and those that make more money have been shown to have less disease. The question: What comes first—health or wealth? Interestingly, we can bring it back to the Belief Circle. Beliefs formed in early childhood affect future potential income. This is why it is so hard for many children raised in a poor or low-income family to rise above their current situation—their belief is "this is the way it is" so their thoughts ruminate on their current circumstances. Emotions such as worthlessness, hopelessness, and sadness have all been found to be higher in lower-income populations. As we have learned, these emotions affect us physically and increase our chances of disease. They have shown healthier people within a certain economic status can work more (take less sick time off from work) and increase their yearly income compared to those dealing with more chronic health issues. These results then flip past limiting beliefs into new empowering beliefs that bring new thoughts, emotions, feelings, actions, and results—improved wealth and health.

Many people have a money belief ceiling. I know this was the case for me several years ago. My husband and I made a good income as physical therapists, but it seemed like no matter how much harder we worked, our income changed little. We had an income goal of $10,000 per month for 20 years. As I moved forward on my exceptional health journey and began investing in myself and flipping my limiting beliefs about my worth, our income increased. In 2014, when we hit our goal, we were ecstatic. Then it was as if we hit a new ceiling. Again, no matter how hard we worked, what we did, little changed regarding our income. It was like we were in this new cycle—yes, a new higher bracket, but the same issue. I believe the belief I had created was, "I'll be happy when we make $10,000 a month." Once we got there, I had some conflicting beliefs (double-mindedness) going on. One thought: I should be content with my current income—my dream income goal—here we were, and I was still looking for joy and happiness. The other thought—I set that goal in my 20s; I am worth more, it's okay to increase the goal and make more money to help more people. Those conflicting beliefs affected my thoughts, my emotions, my feelings about money, and affected my actions—as I would become more successful, I pulled back—going into hiding. My results—this fluctuation kept us at our new "normal"—a financial ceiling.

I know I have been called for exceptional—not normal. I too still have inside work—flipping the penny daily by saying empowering affirmations. I am also increasing my financial skills and money management skills at the same time by investing in coaching and training that helps me put together actions that will bring the results I desire. I get to choose what I believe. I get to put into action what I choose. I have control over my financial health.

Your financial health not only affects you but those you love. Remember, you are setting an example, whether you still have young children at home who are creating beliefs daily or grown children outside the home looking at creating new financial beliefs, your beliefs all the way around the circle to your financial results play a role in future generations. You have control over your financial health.

Go to www.shawnacale.com/book-bonus
Printable Journal Pages and Bonus Resources
to Live an Exceptional Life.

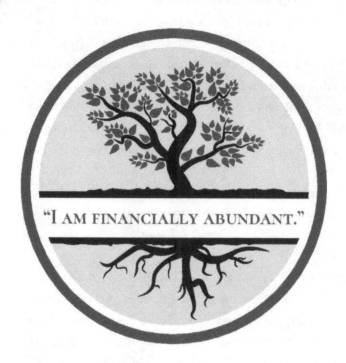

"I AM FINANCIALLY ABUNDANT."

EXERCISE: FINANCIAL GROWTH

1. If your financial health is affecting your overall well-being a great next step is reciting a daily affirmation to flip any limiting money beliefs to empowering money beliefs. You can also add an essential oil along with the affirmation as an anchor.

ENERGY

"The things you do either give you energy or drain you. Choose wisely."
~ Unknown

In 2010, after my 3rd miscarriage in a 10-year period, my energy was drained. I was searching for answers. One stone at a time would appear. I would take a step—my energy returned. I could do what needed to be done, but I wanted more. I wanted the energy to do the things I loved to do with those I loved.

Exceptional had been my beacon for months, and then I woke from my dream—I wrote each letter out—spelling the word ExSEPshNL and then spelling out LIFE. When the Lord gave me the E to LIFE, I knew the ExSEPshNL Formula was the solution to gaining back the energy I so desperately was seeking. I did not understand how much I would learn about energy in the following months and years. My goal of this book was to share with you how the choices I made and the choices you make affect what we have, what we do, and most importantly who we become. Energy is necessary for all three, we are energetic beings.

Energy—just the word itself can bring up so many pictures in our minds. The ExSEPshNL Formula leads to more energy, starting from the powerhouse deep within our mitochondria at the cellular level all the way to the ability for our heart to beat and for us to share our love with others. What I didn't realize for so long is that many of the "normal" choices we make drain our energy levels—what I call energy zappers.

How can you regain your energy and have a vibrant and thriving life? Follow the ExSEPshNL Formula. Start with a positive growth mindset full of gratitude every morning and Ex-It off the roads that have not been leading you where you want to go. Then take the time and Ex-It onto the roads that lead you towards your goals, dreams, and who you were created to become on your journey. Whether you start off your day nice and slow or on the go, you get to write your story.

Here is an example of my exceptional morning, day, and night.

Exceptional Morning Routine (Example- 1 hour)

I begin the day with what I call PMF (prayer, meditation, and fasting). It's my way to fill my cup so I can focus my energy on God and others from a place of abundance instead of overwhelm.

Prayer has been found to light up the brain and whether I am starting my morning relaxed with a time of prayer and my bible devotion or I am ready to get moving and go for a prayer/gratitude walk I have found that prayer energizes me and opens my heart. I start with my morning affirmation: *"I begin this day with love in my heart."* During my prayer time I give praise to God, bless those I love and those that are bothering me and release them. I then think of at least three things I am grateful for that morning, even the hard things. This is also when I grab my essential oils and anoint myself and release any emotions that are no longer serving me as I repeat my affirmation- *"I love myself unconditionally."*

Meditation is a great way to activate the vagus nerve, lower stress and the stress hormone—cortisol, increase blood flow to the brain, and release endorphins for greater energy. I will either do a guided or silent meditation sitting or lying down, or I will do a guided walking meditation and/or focus on scripture or an affirmation. I always start my meditations with 2-5 minutes of deep breathing, along with an essential oil.

Fasting is also part of my exceptional mornings. My goal is always to have my breakfast (breaking the fast) 12-16 hours after my last meal. Fasting allows the body to stay in the parasympathetic mode "rest, digest and heal" and allows me to have better blood sugar regulation, hormonal balance, and the energy and focus I need to start my day.

Exceptional Day Routine (Example 8-12 hours)

I review my Exceptional Roadmap, which is where I keep my information on the goals I am working towards and the direction I choose to move in my life to live out my purpose on purpose. I then follow my daily schedule in my planner (paper or online) to keep me focused and on task with the commitments I have set with others and myself. When I find myself on rabbit trails, I will use the affirmation: "I am self-disciplined." I invest in others and choose business endeavors that bring finances into my home to support my family. I choose FOOD to nourish and energize me and have a water routine that keeps me on track to drink 8 glasses or more a day.

Exceptional Evening Routine (Example 1-2 hours)

I end the day much like I begin the day (filling my cup)—a walk, reading, a hot bath, time alone to unwind, or time with family and/or friends to reconnect. I anoint myself with oils and release the stressors of the day by reviewing my day and letting go of emotions that are no longer serving me. I ask God to forgive me for any sins I have committed, and I forgive myself for mistakes and imperfections. I crawl into bed at a time that allows me to have 8 hours of sleep and rest and recharge for another exceptional day.

EX-IT'S

Ex-It Plan #1: Exit the Normal Road of Excuses.

Ex-It Plan #2: Be an Example.

Ex-It Plan #3: Exercise

Go to www.shawnacale.com/book-bonus
Printable Journal Pages and Bonus Resources
to Live an Exceptional Life.

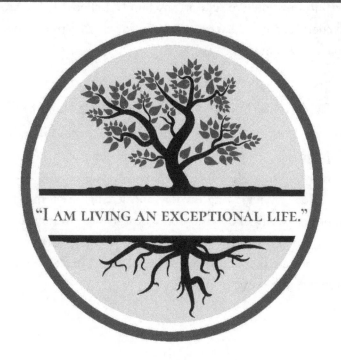

"I AM LIVING AN EXCEPTIONAL LIFE."

EXERCISE: ENERGY

1. You have written your story. Now it's time to write your roadmap to your exceptional life. Start with writing your morning routine and making it a new habit.

2. Life no longer gets in your way of living a healthy lifestyle because you know the Ex-Its you can take. Write your exceptional day routine and live it out.

3. How you end your day will help you tomorrow. Remember, you are worthy of an exceptional life and you get to choose how to end your day—write what it looks like guiding you nightly.

EXCEPTIONAL ROAD MAP

ExSEPshNL Solution: Take Responsibility for Your Life

ExSEPshNL Formula: First Step—Walk

ExSEPshNL Solution: Unconditional Love

ExSEPshNL Formula: Next Step—Love Yourself Unconditionally.

ExSEPshNL Solution: Freedom

ExSEPshNL Formula: Next Step—Forgiveness.

ExSEPshNL Solution: Less Stress

ExSEPshNL Formula: Next Step—Deep Breathing.

ExSEPshNL Solution: Hormonal Balance

ExSEPshNL Formula: Next Step—Sleep, Hydrate and Nourish.

ExSEPshNL Solution: More Energy

ExSEPshNL Formula: Last Step—Live an Exceptional Life.

LAST STEP

I have enjoyed our walk and talk. I hope you have learned what you need to move forward in your life. As I shared in My Story—trauma can often set up limiting beliefs (lies) that we believe for way too long. If you too have had trauma, there is hope.

Have you taken the first step—walking? I want to challenge you right now to pick up your mat and walk. I have found when you take this one step it leads you down the exceptional road and you find taking the next step a little easier. You may say at this point. "Shawna thanks, I know I should do these things, but who has the time and energy to do them? Not Me!" I get it. I have been there and felt that way too. Remember, I didn't even know where to start, how to start, or if I could start. I needed help. I also knew I had a choice. I could either continue going down the path I was going, which was not serving me AT ALL. Or I could choose to take baby steps to walk down a different path and live a different life. I knew God gave me the ExSEPshNL Formula, but staying on the exceptional road has not always felt possible. What I learned through the process—I had to let go of perfection and the fear of failure and have faith to take the next step, no matter the outcome. If I fell down, I learned from the fall and would get up and take another step. You can do the same—TAKE ONE STEP—when you fall down, it's okay. Learn from the fall, get up, and take another step.

"But Shawna, I already have a list of diseases. It's too late for me." Living an exceptional life is not about your past—it's about your today and your tomorrow. You may not receive a cure, but I promise if you put the ExSEPshNL Formula into effect you will see change, if not on the outside on the inside. Each of these solutions has been scientifically proven again and again because they work.

Change for me was difficult, and it may not be easy for you. I mean change takes a lot of energy, the energy I didn't have. But here's what happened: I implemented change one by one and my life improved within 30 days of deciding enough was enough. With each step, I had a little less stress and was feeling good. I mean really good. Such as not yelling at my kids kind of good. Going to the park, planting flowers, racing my kids in the swimming pool, good. I was beginning to no longer live the "normal" life, the life I was told by the doctors was just how it is for us momma's—tired, worn-out, overwhelmed—the life I had accepted for too long. My life was changing, I was changing. I was living an exceptional life. A life filled with energy and purpose. Start small. Take a 5-minute walk today and increase it by 5 minutes until you reach the 30-minute mark. Grab your kids, your spouse, a friend, the dog, and take them along if you need to. Put on your earbuds or headphones and turn on a podcast or listen to some music. Whatever brings you joy and/or motivates you to take the first step. Grab yourself a bottle of water too. Let your family know you are committed to taking care of yourself so you can better take care of them. I promise they love you and they want you to be happy and healthy. Guess what? When you have more energy, they won't even notice all that you are doing for yourself daily because they will be so excited you have the time and energy to invest in them too.

I would love for you to let me know what reading this book has done for you. I am here to cheer you on, answer questions, and even be that person you want to prove wrong. You've got this!

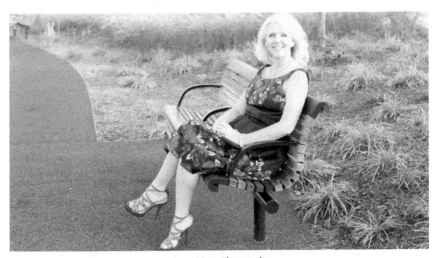

Sonja Marie Photography

12

Winning Results-
Testimonies

*"If you're brave enough to say goodbye,
life will reward you with a new hello."*
~ Paul Coelho

God gave me the ExSEPshNL Formula as a gift to give to others. He never meant for me to hold unto it for myself or to put up on a shelf never to use. I had to say goodbye to fear of what others would think to write this book. I hope you have found it to be a gift—a smile, a hello from a friend. Thank you for taking the time to read it and to put the challenges, actions, and exercises into motion and see change.

I have known since I was a little girl that my purpose was to help others with their health. As a child, I thought I was going to be a doctor. In high school, I realized my calling was to be a physical therapist and a mom. With time, my calling has morphed into this wonderful passion of serving women ready for change and holistic health. I am grateful that each part of my story has led me right here to where I am today. Here to serve you.

This is where the Belief Circle ends and begins. When you see results, it locks in your belief. When you have winning results, it locks in these empowering beliefs that bring these wonderful positive thoughts, kind words and your cells multiply and flourish, your emotions bring this flood of happy chemicals that cover every part of your body and you send out your love to the world, you feel better than ever; you do actions that bring you holistic health and the winning results just keep coming.

When you spend almost 10 years writing a book, you have lots of information. I knew all of it could not go into this book, so a coach recommended I dive deeper and put together an online course along with a group coaching program to help women meet their health goals—since that is my specialty. It was like I went back in time to January 2012 when I did my first ExSEPshNL Health program with a few women through Facebook and emails. I've grown a lot since then and my program has become a way to invest in women ready to invest in themselves, and it has become more wonderful and exciting than I could have ever imagined—and I dream big.

The women who took part in my first 10- week Exceptional Health Masterclass were such an inspiration. I knew I had to finish this book for them and all the other women waiting for the ExSEPshNL Formula.

This is their story. Their winning results.
Their personal testimonies.

Each of them took the challenge, completed their mission and are now less stressed, feel better, and have more energy to do the things they love to do.

Exceptional Women Living an Exceptional Life.

EXERCISE

"I knew I needed to exercise, but I thought I didn't have the time."
~ Monica

About a month before starting the masterclass, I experienced a sudden onset of panic/anxiety attacks. This was something I had never experienced before. I felt like I was out of control of my own body and life. I really wanted to get to the root of the cause of this issue, but my family physician just wanted to give me this pill or that pill and wasn't worried about what caused my problems. About a year before this onset of anxiety, I had an acute diverticulitis attack which put me in the hospital for a few days. I knew my gut was not healthy at all! I was overweight, had poor gut health & diverticulosis, felt exhausted all the time, had insomnia, stressed to the max (but really didn't realize it because that was my 'normal'), my hormones were all out of whack, I had multiple vitamin deficiencies, as well as, deficiencies of numerous neurotransmitters. I knew I needed to get healthier so I could do a better job at taking care of all that was required of me as a home manager/mom.

I joined the Exceptional Health Masterclass (EHM) and knew I was all in because something needed to change in my life for me to get better. I had already changed my diet pretty dramatically by going vegan, so hydration and nutrition were not a big issue for me. So how did this EHM change my life? First of all, and I think most importantly, it got me moving! I knew I needed to exercise, but thought I didn't have the time. In reality, I had the time, I just didn't prioritize exercise. I am a mom to five amazing children... an adult son who still lives at home, pre-teen twin boys, a teenage daughter, and our youngest daughter, which requires a bit more of mommy as she has some special needs. My life is 'BUSY'! I now make time daily to move my body in some form. Whether it is a walk with the family all together, yoga, or Pilates, I am moving daily! Secondly, it helped me to see how important it was to bring my emotional, spiritual, and physical entities of my life together. We are emotional, spiritual, and physical beings, so we must support all these areas. The affirmations, emotional release technique, and the meditation/deep breathing alongside the exercise helped me tremendously over this course to help me completely eliminate my anxiety, lose 10lbs (which wasn't originally part of my goal, but hey, love that I lost weight!), I have more energy, sleep better, and feel like I am the mom/wife I am supposed to be to my children and husband. My eyes were opened to how important it was for me to care for myself and do so without feeling guilty!

Biggest Transformation: Anxiety was lowered—YES!
Biggest Takeaway: Get moving!

SPIRITUAL

"It is an amazing feeling to know I can and I did."
~ Susie

I was overwhelmed with anxiety and depression caused by Parkinson's. The meds were causing me to gain weight, which only led to more frustration and depression. I knew I wanted off the roller coaster that my spiritual, emotional, and physical self was on but I didn't know-how. I knew I needed someone to talk to. But who? One day I saw a post about an Exceptional Health Masterclass. It intrigued me. I thought it would be a class about losing weight and debated about 10 minutes with myself before signing up. It wasn't till the second week of class that I realized this wasn't just about weight. It was about your 'Why'. It was about getting off the roller coaster and taking the exit to a life that is exceptional. These last 3 months have been a journey of flipping limited beliefs and learning how to take time to work on just 'ME'. I attended all the classes and completed all the homework because I wanted a change. I lost my minimum goal of 10 lbs but I gained so much more in learning from Shawna. She gave us the tools to make a roadmap to work on our next goal as we continue to live an exceptional life. I can never thank her enough for her encouragement to make the jump off the roller coaster and say I CAN. Overwhelmed, anxiety and depression aren't in my vocabulary anymore because I'm a winner. Thanks, Shawna, for leading us down the ExSEPshNL road.

Biggest Takeaway: I'm worth it because I'm a winner.
Goal: To lose 10 lbs by my 65th birthday—Goal Met!

EMOTIONAL

"I have been working on my limited beliefs and releasing trapped emotions and it has been amazing at how it has changed all aspects of my life."
~ Rose

I was having an anger issue; I wasn't sure what to do with all this overload. It affected everything that I did. I joined the Exceptional Health Masterclass and learned that it was a hidden emotion since I was a year old and not feeling loved. I have been working on my limiting beliefs and releasing trapped emotions, and it has been amazing how it has changed all aspects of my life.

Biggest Transformation: Emotionally—able to handle living.
Biggest Takeaway: That I have choices in everything I do.

PHYSICAL

"I became aware of what my body needs, and to listen and trust my instinct."
~ Teresa

Before the Exceptional Health Masterclass (EHM) I had given up on losing weight. I had failed at many attempts. I was not sure I could make the changes. I joined EHM, and I learned to flip the negative thoughts. I became aware of what my body needs, and to listen and trust my instinct. I have participated in other classes taught by Shawna and was always pleased with the overall results. I actually lost 20 lbs in 10 weeks and have a plan to keep it off and reach my stretch goal of 40 lbs lost for good.

Biggest Takeaway: I am a winner, and I can accomplish anything that I choose to accomplish.
Affirmation: "I love myself unconditionally."

SLEEP

"Learning that small things all together can make big differences."
~ Penny

When I began the Exceptional Health Masterclass I was having hip pain from an injury sustained while running a 5K six-plus years prior, along with adrenal, sleep, and inability to lose weight issues. I had just come off of hip surgery two months prior to this class and was starting to suspect that the surgery didn't resolve my hip pain. I was in a state of complete frustration. I joined the Exceptional Health Masterclass and learned so many of my issues were directly related to my hip pain. Once I discovered this and started using the tools, I was being taught I discovered that making conscious choices in my daily life would improve my state of mind and wellbeing to a point that was easily managed. I was able to get restorative sleep that improved my adrenals and by the end of the class had lost a total of 12 lbs. What a blessing Shawna and this class have been to me and I look forward to continuing doing the little things to make big differences!

Biggest Transformation: Organizational skills—alleviate stress.
Affirmation: "I am self-disciplined."

HYDRATION

"I've identified several areas in my health that I can begin making small changes for even greater support."
~ Alicia

This journey has been wonderful. I had low energy, along with morning fog and fatigue. After starting the program, I became properly hydrated. I started realizing the importance of sleep and using a nightly protocol according to my chronotype. I began walking every day and using that time to reflect, pray, and be grateful. I started deep breathing and using my oils daily to release stress and emotions. I started to make a conscious effort to choose nutrient-dense foods instead of packing in empty calories. I continued daily praying and reading my bible. I realized I am currently living out my God-given purpose and I'm extremely fulfilled. I am investing my resources in my family, my community, and my business. I've identified several areas in my health that I can begin making small changes for even greater support. I am taking vitamins and supplements to support every system in my body.

As a result of the class, I have been able to wake up with no brain fog, and with no alarm clock by 7 am. My morning fatigue has completely disappeared. I have energy 10/10. After I introduced nutrient-dense foods, (week 9 and 10) I found I lost my taste for processed desserts/sweets. I am enjoying my newfound levels of energy and will continue my weight loss journey to lose another 5 pounds. Thank you, Shawna! You poured so much into us throughout this program and it has blessed many lives.

Biggest Transformation: *Energy*

Biggest Takeaway: *Being full is not as important as being truly filled with the nutrients and hydration my body needs.*

NUTRITION

"Learning more about what foods to eat and why they are helpful or not helpful to my body, health, weight, emotions."
~ Johnna

I have tried a lot of diets over the years, and lost some weight, but gained it back in a few weeks to a few months. Tired and emotional a lot. Learning more about what food to eat and why these foods are helpful or not helpful to my body, health, weight, emotions. I have learned a lot about how much my emotions and stress and spiritual life have been a big part of my weight and energy and overall health. I knew some things we learned but did not put a lot of them into practice and everyday life. Knowledge doesn't help if you don't use it. Shawna helps us see how important it all is and like a puzzle (I bought one at a garage sale one time and we worked on it and at the end, one piece was missing, so disappointing all those hours of work and 1 piece made all our work not complete) I never buy puzzles at garage sales anymore... LOL!) or even a Jenga game, with missing parts it all falls apart. Or like Matt. 7:24-27, a house built on the rock will stand, but on sand, without a strong foundation, it can not stand the rains and winds. And everyone's life has rain, storms and winds, different ones and different times. And if you get stuck or can't get over it, you can't grow and learn from it. Limiting beliefs to empowering beliefs. The class helped me in several areas and now I have a better foundation and information and tools in my belt to help me, and have grown and learned a lot and still have a long way to go. As a Christian, I love how Shawna brings the bible verses and scripture and affirmations into the lessons. But I think it is shared with so much love and compassion to help others, where everyone can learn and grow from it.

Loved the class and would recommend it to anyone wanting to be healthier, happier, and losing weight is the extra bonus.

Biggest transformation: Stress was a big part and learning to see it, deal with it, work through it better.

End Result: Feeling better and now know how I can be healthier and eat better and lose weight.

LIFE

"The tools I have learned to utilize in EHM is allowing me to see that I can get my health/blood glucose under control."

~ Rindi

I have been a type 2 diabetic for 20 years. I can honestly say that I have been in denial a lot of that time. I went through diabetic classes when I was first diagnosed and again 2 years ago. I felt like everything I learned from the classes was the "cookie-cutter" plan, the same treatment for everyone. I really believed there was more than that and the EHM showed me there is. The opportunity to join the EHM was one I didn't want to pass up. God told me to love myself and invest in my health. I learned there is more to taking care of myself than just diet and exercise. Our emotional and spiritual health is vitally important too. Releasing stored emotions and limiting beliefs plays an important part in getting my physical health back in control. I am taking my limiting belief of "I have no choices" and flipping that belief to "I do have choices." The tools I have learned to utilize in EHM is allowing me to see that I can get my health/blood glucose under control. I am currently searching for a functional medicine doctor to work with me in my journey to dig deeper into seeing what my specific treatment should be and eventually getting off medication.

Biggest Transformation: Self-Disciplined
Biggest Takeaway: There is more to life than the normal path!

LIFE
"I did know that I could not lose weight."
~ Rhenea

Before I started EHM I was having problems with hormones, inability to lose weight, lack of sleep, fatigue, and joint pain. I didn't even realize I was having some of these problems because they had just become the norm for me. I did know that I could not lose weight. I had already tried everything, so my mind was already against me. By being in this Masterclass, one of the first things I learned was that I had to break that mindset. I was given the skill set to not only break through this barrier but to be able to use the same skills to break other limiting beliefs. I not only could lose weight, I did. Thirteen pounds. And that is just the start.

Goal: To lose weight and resolve other health issues to be able to live a healthy life.
Biggest Takeaway: That I can. And I will. I am empowered to change and to take control.

I Am a Winner

Today, I realized I am a winner
I felt I should stand up and say
My name is... and I am a winner!

But in today's world
We are taught to hide our inner achievements
Fear of pride keeps us quiet

Those limiting beliefs are what kept me stuck
But flipping that penny and seeing the other side
Left me feeling better than ever before

It started with just the occasional good job
Or maybe you got this, go girl
Then it became a daily affirmation
To appreciate all the hard work I had done

Then it was more of a habit
Something to say when the road looked too difficult

My habit became easier each day
It became a daily desire, a need
I was no longer a loser, a failure, not enough
Because I was a winner, a success,
I was enough

Then I was ready to tell the world
Show them the new me
Today, I would announce

I am a winner!

The freedom it brought
The joy inside was more
Then I ever thought

Now you may be saying
Good for you!
That could never be me

I don't amount to anything
Just ask anyone to see

I thought the same
Feelings of worthlessness
And wanting to run far away

But someone gave me hope
Told me I was worthy
And to just say the words

You see if you wait to feel
Like you are the winner you are
With the thoughts, I am not
Then you will stay where you are

It's just 4 words, "I am a winner"
I can do anything
I wish I could say, It's easy to do
Taking that first step, Is always the hardest

But the feeling it brings
The actions you will see
The results that will be
Will bring the empowering belief
You are a winner too!

I wrote this poem to the Exceptional Women of the first Graduation Exceptional Health Masterclass in May 2020. This poem was based on my "I am an Addict" poem I wrote in October 2010. These exceptional women inspired me so much using the *Flip the Penny Principle I* decided it was time to do the same—I am no longer an addict. I am a winner!

Go to www.shawnacale.com/winner
Leave your transformational testimony
so we can celebrate with you.

Join Our Exceptional Health Masterclass:

YOUR MISSION,

SHOULD YOU CHOOSE TO ACCEPT IT,

IS TO CREATE, IMPLEMENT AND REACH YOUR

HEALTH GOAL IN THE EXCEPTIONAL HEALTH

MASTERCLASS IN 10-WEEKS OR LESS,

SO YOU CAN BE LESS STRESSED, FEEL BETTER,

AND HAVE MORE ENERGY.

AND WE'LL BE DOING IT TOGETHER,

WITH CLARITY, DIRECTION,

AND LOVING SUPPORT EVERY STEP OF THE WAY.

25% OFF Masterclass promo code: hello
www.shawnacale.com/ehm

Notes

Introduction:

1. Dave Jenkins, "What is the Meaning of Dunamis in the Bible?"
   https://www.christianity.com/wiki/christian-terms/what-is-
   the-meaning-of-dunamis-in-the-bible.html

Chapter 1

1. Louis Haber, *Women Pioneers of Science,* (New York, NY: Har-
   court Brace Jovanovich, 1979)
2. Stacey Kelly, "The Impact of Early Years on a Child's Future."
   https://www.earlyyearsstorybox.com/impact-early-years-
   childs-future/

Chapter 2

1. Stephen A. Robinson, "Do the emotional side-effects of con-
   traceptives come from pharmacological or psychological
   mechanisms." https://pubmed.ncbi.nlm.nih.gov/15236788/
2. Bill Phillips, *Body for Life: 12 Weeks to Mental and Physical
   Strength* (New York, NY: HarperCollins Publishers, 1999)

Chapter 3

1. Richard Lenti, "70% of American's on Prescription Drugs." http://nationalpainreport.com/70-of-americans-on-prescription-drugs-8820549.html
2. Jordan Reubin, *The Maker's Diet: The 40-Day Health Experience That Will Change Your Life Forever (Lake Mary, FL: Siloam Press, 2004)*

Chapter 4

1. See Exodus 4:10
2. See Genesis 18:12
3. MJ Shield, "Anti-inflammatory drugs and their effects on cartilage synthesis and renal function." https://pubmed.ncbi.nlm.nih.gov/7821339/
4. David Stewart, *Healing Oils of the Bible* (Marble Hill, MO: Care Publications, 2003)
5. Young Living Essential Oils is who I bought my first Premium Starter Kit through and the only oil company I trust. Member #1249570.
6. Raindrop and Aromatherapy Defined: https://www.raindrop-training.com/programs/CCI/definitions.shtml
7. Care Intensives Defined: https://www.raindroptraining.com/programs/intensive.shtml
8. Carolyn L. Mein, D.C., *Releasing Emotional Patterns with Essential Oils* (Rancho Santa Fe, CA: visionary Press, 1998)

Chapter 5

1. Septuagint: https://en.m.wikipedia.org/wiki/Septuagint
2. See Matthew 18:21-22
3. *American Book of Philology Vol. XXVII, Greek and Latin Etymolo-*

gies Pg 308. https://www.journals.uchicago.edu/doi/pdf/10.1086/ 360233

4. CDC Prevention Programs: https://www.heart.org/en/get-involved/advocate/federal-priorities/cdc-prevention-programs#

5. Stephen M. Rappaport, "Genetic Factors Are Not the Major Causes of Chronic Diseases." https://www.ncbi.nlm.nih.gov/pmc/articles/PMC4841510/

Chapter 6

1. J Vina, "Exercise acts as a drug; the pharmacological benefits of exercise." https://www.ncbi.nlm.nih.gov/pmc/articles/PMC3448908/

2. Harold G. Koenig, "Religion, Spirituality, and Health: The Research and Clinical Implications." https://www.ncbi.nlm.nih.gov/pmc/articles/PMC3671693/

3. Glenn Berkenkamp, "Treat Yourself to a Gratitude Walk," https://gratefulness.org/resource/treat-yourself-to-an-immune-boosting-mood-elevating-gratitude-walk/

Chapter 7

1. Thought. (n.d.). In Lexico Powered by *Oxford English dictionary*. Retrieved from https://www.lexico.com/definition/thought#h69891057025300

2. Cedarwood tree: https://treesymbolism.com/cedar-tree-tymbolism-meaning.html

3. Caroline Leaf, *Who Switched Off My Brain? : Controlling Toxic Thoughts and Emotions*, (Dallas TX: Switch On Your Brain, 2009)

4. Caroline Leaf: *Switch On Your Brain: The Key to Peak Happiness, Thinking, and Health*, (Grand Rapids, Michigan: Baker Books, 2013)

5. Alexander Loyd, *The Healing Code*, (Peoria, AZ: Intermedia Publishing Group, Inc., 2010)

Chapter 8

1. Candace B.Pert Ph.D. *Molecules of Emotion.* (New York, New York: Scribner, 1997)
2. Caroline Leaf: *Switch On Your Brain: The Key to Peak Happiness, Thinking, and Health*, (Grand Rapids, Michigan: Baker Books, 2013)
3. Daniel Goleman, *Emotional Intelligence.* (New York, NY: Bantam Books, 1997)
4. Lauri Nummenmaa, *Bodily maps of emotions.* (Proceedings of the National Academy of Sciences Jan 2014, 111 (2) 646-651) https://www.pnas.org/content/111/2/646
5. 6 seconds: https://www.6seconds.org/2019/06/19/why-six-seconds-about-our-intriguing-name/
6. Kathryn K. Ridout, "Adverse Childhood Experiences Run Deep: Toxic Early Life Stress, Telomeres, and Mitochondrial DNA Copy Number, the Biological Markers of Cumulative Stress." https://pubmed.ncbi.nlm.nih.gov/30067291/
7. ACEs Quiz: See https://www.safelaunch.org/aces-quiz/
8. Anxiety: See https://finds.life.church/change-your-perspective-anxiety/
9. Donna Bach, ND, "Clinical EFT (Emotional Freedom Techniques) Improves Multiple Physiological Markers of Health." https://www.ncbi.nlm.nih.gov/pmc/articles/PMC6381429/
10. See https://www.tappingsolutionfoundation.org/science-and-research/
11. See https://www.tappingsolutionfoundation.org/
12. Tapping Video: See https://www.youtube.com/watch?v=pAclBdj2oZU&feature=youtu.be
13. Kelly Brogan, Change Your Food Heal Your Mood E-Book:

https://kellybroganmd.com/wp-content/uploads/2016/01/ChangeYourFoodHealYourMoodEBook.pdf

14. Kelly Brogan, *A Mind of Your Own: The Truth About Depression and How Women Can Heal Their Bodies to Reclaim Their Lives.* (New York, NY: Harper Wave, 2016)

15. See The American Institute of Stress https://www.stress.org/42-worrying-workplace-stress-statistics#

16. Stephen W Porges. *The Polyvagal Theory: Neurophysiological Foundations of Emotions, attachment, communication, and self-regulation.* (New York, NY: W.W. Norton & Co, Inc., 2011)

17. Bradley Nelson, *The Emotion Code.* (New York, NY: St. Martin's Press, 2019)

18. Disillusioned (n.d). In Lexico Powered by Oxford English dictionary. Retrieved from https://www.lexico.com/definition/disillusioned

19. Caroline Leaf: *Switch On Your Brain: the Key to Peak Happiness, Thinking, and Health,* (Grand Rapids, Michigan: Baker Books, 2013)

20. Loren Toussaint, *Effects of lifetime stress exposure on mental and physical health in young adulthood: How stress degrades and forgiveness protects health, J Health Psychol 2016 Jun;21(6):1004-14. doi: 10.1177/1359105314544132. Epub 2014 Aug 19. https://pubmed.ncbi.nlm.nih.gov/25139892/*

Chapter 9

1. Simon Sinek, *Start with Why: How Great Leaders Inspire Everyone to Take Action,* (New York, NY: Penguin Group, 2009)

2. Ted Talk: See https://www.ted.com/talks/simon_sinek_how_great_leaders_inspire_action?language=en

3. Elizabeth Lipski, *Digestion Connection: The Simple, Natural Plan to Combat Diabetes, Heart Disease, Osteoporosis, Arthritis, Acid Reflux—and More!* (New York, NY: Rodale, 2013)

4. Kelly Brogan, *A Mind of Your Own: The Truth About Depression and How Women Can Heal Their Bodies to Reclaim Their Lives.* (New York, NY: Harper Wave, 2016)

5. Valerie Saxion, *Every Body Has Parasites: If You're Alive, You're at Risk!* (Minneapolis, MN: Bronze Bow Publishing, Inc., 2003)

6. Megan Clapp, "*Gut microbiota's effect on mental health: The gut-brain axis*" Clin Pract. 2017 Sep 15; 7(4): 987. https://www.ncbi.nlm.nih.gov/pmc/articles/PMC5641835/#

7. Henry W. Wright, *A More Excellent Way to Be in Health,* (New Kensington, PA: Whitaker House, 2009)

8. H.M. Kim, "*Lavender oil inhibits immediate-type allergic reaction in mice and rats*", *J Pharm Pharmacol 1999 Feb;51(2):221-6. doi: 10.1211/0022357991772178. https://pubmed.ncbi.nlm.nih.gov/10217323*

9. Li-Wei Chien, Su Li Cheng, Chi Feng Liu, "*The Effect of Lavender Aromatherapy on Autonomic Nervous System in Midlife Women with Insomnia*". *Evidence-Based Complementary and Alternative Medicine, vol. 2012 Article ID 740813, 8 pages, 2012. https://doi.org/10.1155/2012/740813*

10. Carolyn L. Mein, D.C., *Releasing Emotional Patterns with Essential Oils* (Rancho Santa Fe, CA: VisionWare Press, 1998)

11. See https://shawnacale.com/lavender

12. RK Naviaux, "*Metabolic features of the cell danger response.*" Mitochondrion. 2014 May;16:7-17. doi: 10.1016/j.mito.2013.08.006. Epub 2013 Aug 24. PMID: 23981537. https://pubmed.ncbi.nlm.nih.gov/23981537/

13. Raindrop: https://www.raindroptraining.com/programs/CCI/definitions.shtml

14. JA Woods, KR Wilund, SA Martin, BM Kistler, "*Exercise, inflammation and aging.*" *Aging Dis. 2012;3(1):130-140.* https://www.ncbi.nlm.nih.gov/pmc/articles/PMC3320801/

15. Suzanne M de la Monte, and Jack R Wands. "Alzheimer's disease is type 3 diabetes-evidence reviewed." *Journal of diabetes science and technology* vol. 2,6 (2008): 1101-13. doi:10.1177/

193229680800200619. https://www.ncbi.nlm.nih.gov/pmc/articles/PMC2769828/

16. L Stojanovich, D Marisavljevich. "Stress as a trigger of autoimmune disease." Autoimmun Rev. 2008 Jan;7(3):209-13. doi: 10.1016/j.autrev.2007.11.007. Epub 2007 Nov 29. PMID: 18190880. https://pubmed.ncbi.nlm.nih.gov/18190880/

17. Jessica Robinson-Papp, et al. "Vagal dysfunction and small intestinal bacterial overgrowth: novel pathways to chronic inflammation in HIV." *AIDS (London, England)* vol. 32,9 (2018): 1147-1156. doi:10.1097/QAD.0000000000001802. https://www.ncbi.nlm.nih.gov/pmc/articles/PMC5945300/

18. Coffee Enemas: See https://www.upyoursjava.com

Chapter 10

1. David Nutt, et al. "Sleep disorders as core symptoms of depression." *Dialogues in clinical neuroscience* vol. 10,3 (2008): 329-36. doi:10.31887/DCNS.2008.10.3/dnutt. https://www.ncbi.nlm.nih.gov/pmc/articles/PMC3181883/

2. See https://www.consumerreports.org/sleep/why-americans-cant-sleep/

3. Peir Hossein Koulivand, et al. "Lavender and the nervous system." *Evidence-based complementary and alternative medicine : eCAM* vol. 2013 (2013): 681304. doi:10.1155/2013/681304. *https://www.ncbi.nlm.nih.gov/pmc/articles/PMC3612440/*

4. F Batmanghelidj, *Your Bodies Many Cries for Water* (Falls Church, VA: Global Health Solutions, 1995)

5. Jordan Reubin, *The Maker's Diet: The 40-Day Health Experience That Will Change Your Life Forever (Lake Mary, FL: Siloam Press, 2004)*

6. Nicole M Avena, et al. "Evidence for sugar addiction: behavioral and neurochemical effects of intermittent, excessive sugar intake." *Neuroscience and biobehavioral reviews* vol. 32,1

(2008): 20-39. doi:10.1016/j.neubiorev.2007.04.019, https://www.ncbi.nlm.nih.gov/pmc/articles/PMC2235907/

7. A Johnstone, "Fasting for weight loss: an effective strategy or latest dieting trend?" Int J Obes (Lond). 2015 May;39(5):727-33. doi: 10.1038/ijo.2014.214. Epub 2014 Dec 26. PMID: 25540982. https://pubmed.ncbi.nlm.nih.gov/25540982/

8. Alessio Nencioni, et al. "Fasting and cancer: molecular mechanisms and clinical application." *Nature reviews. Cancer*vol. 18,11 (2018): 707-719. doi:10.1038/s41568-018-0061-0, https://www.ncbi.nlm.nih.gov/pmc/articles/PMC6938162/

9. Catherine R Marinac, et al. "Prolonged Nightly Fasting and Breast Cancer Prognosis." *JAMA oncology* vol. 2,8 (2016): 1049-55. doi:10.1001/jamaoncol.2016.0164, https://www.ncbi.nlm.nih.gov/pmc/articles/PMC4982776/

10. Lee Bueno, *Fast Your Way to Health* (New Kensington, PA: Whitaker House Publishing, 1991)

11. Jason Fung, Jimmy Moore, *The Complete Guide to Fasting* (Las Vegas, NV: Victory Belt Publishing, 2016)

Chapter 11

1. See https://www.smh.com.au/lifestyle/why-purposeful-people-are-likely-to-live-longer-20140827-1099fz.html

2. Helen Keller, *The Story of My Life*, (New York, NY: Double day Page & Company, 1905)

3. Christine Carter, "What We Get When We Give," Greater Good Magazine: Science-Based Insights for a Meaningful Life. (February 18, 2010) https://greatergood.berkeley.edu/article/item/what_we_get_when_we_give

4. Sophie Bethune, "Money stress weighs on Americans' health," American Psychological Association. (April 2015, Vol 46, No. 4) https://www.apa.org/monitor/2015/04/money-stress

CPSIA information can be obtained
at www.ICGtesting.com
Printed in the USA
LVHW021122120221
679116LV00004B/903